RESEARCH AND RECIPES
ON DEMENTIA, HEART DISEASE,
OSTEOPOROSIS & CANCER

RESEARCH AND RECIPES ON DEMENTIA, HEART DISEASE, OSTEOPOROSIS & CANCER

BY

ROSEMARY C. FISHER

WARREN H. GREEN, INC.
St. Louis, Missouri, U.S.A.

Published by

WARREN H. GREEN, INC.
8356 Olive Boulevard
Saint Louis, Missouri 63132 U.S.A.

ISBN NO. 0-87527-518-4

Printed in the United States of America

DEDICATION

This book is dedicated to the memory of my husband, Alvin I. Fisher.
October 1, 1917 - December 22, 1994

In June, 1994, my husband was diagnosed with possible Alzheimer's disease and Multi-infarct disease. He died December, 1994, six months later.

Previous to his June diagnosis, he had had no indication of any kind of dementia. In March, 1994, my husband had had a colonoscopy. His report showed only that he had grade 2 internal hemorrhoids. Also noted on the report was that the gastroenterologist thanked the cardiologist "for the opportunity to participate in this pleasant gentleman's care." There was no mention of any symptoms of dementia at that time. Any symptoms of dementia my husband may have had previous to his diagnosis would have been classified as "Oh that's part of aging." His life was productive until the time he entered the hospital in June due to an accident with his foot.

After his death in December, the summary on my husband's autopsy came as a shock. He was described as having had Alzheimer's disease, Multi-infarct disease and Binswanger's disease. All were diagnosed as severe. Though I had been told after he entered the hospital that he had some form of Alzheimer's and Multi-infarct disease, I'd not heard about Binswanger's disease. Binswanger's disease (also called incephalitis subcorticalis chronica) is a sub cortical progressive deterioration of mental capacity without clear focal neurologic symptoms.

When I tried to understand how he could have had such advanced dementias and not shown the more severe symptoms, I looked at his diet (which had changed dramatically once he entered the hospital). Our diet was a low-fat, high mineral content diet. This, no doubt, had an effect in allowing my husband to live a normal life longer than ever would been expected for one with his types of severe dementia. His attending neurologists agreed.

After realizing this, I decided to share the research and recipes upon which my husband's diet was based. My hope in writing this book is to help even one person slow the progession of these diseases, and if the diet is started at an early age, to help even one person prevent their onset.

As in my previous books, all proceeds derived from the sale of this book will be given to organizations working directly with the poor or to the poor themselves. This is my way to "Thank God" for helping me to reverse osteoporosis in myself and for helping my husband to have just 6 months of debilitation with severe dementia instead of years.

A TRIBUTE

This book is also dedicated to the memory of **Warren H. Green, publisher.** Warren, along with his wife, Joyce, dedicated his life to getting the written word to "you."

Many of your lives, I am sure, have been changed because of his dedication. Without the written word, you would not have the knowledge that would allow you to make changes in your lifestyle that would benefit your bodies. It is not how *long* we live, but the *quality* of life we have in living.

May you be blessed and remember Warren and his dedication to making this knowledge available to you.

ACKNOWLEDGEMENTS

I would like to express my deep appreciation to my daughter-in-law, Joyce M. DeHaan, M.A., M.A., and to my son, Gerard E. Fisher, Ph.D., for their loving support and assistance in the preparation of this book and my other books, without whom this project would never have been completed. Joyce's long days of effort in the final editing process have contributed immensely to the book's effectiveness. I will always be in her debt.

I would also like to thank Robert A. Heinle, M.D., for his support and encouragement to me throughout the years to continue my research and writing. I also want to thank Sally Marlowe, N.P., Director of Arthritis Pain Treatment Center in Clearwater, Florida. Sally measured my bone density on her mobile unit called DEXA, making it possible to document my progress in increasing and maintaining by bone density. Later, she, with Dr. Dale Braman, presented my osteoporosis case of increasing bone density after the age of 70 as an outstanding case study at the AHPA Convention (December 3, 1988) in Tampa, Florida. Furthermore, she has been an unwavering source of inspiration and assistance.

For reviewing my manuscript, I especially appreciate the efforts of Robert A. Heinle, M.D., and John A. O'Sullivan, M.D.

Among the many others who have provided years of support, encouragement, ideas and research assistance to me are Jessie Uy, M.S., M.B.A., Marie Bresson, M.S.R.N., and Barbara Heinle.

My lasting appreciation for all your help.

FOREWORD

I first met Rosemary Fisher In September 1976 when her husband, Al, was hospitalized with a sudden heart attack. The heart attack was a rather large one and one of the three major arteries to the heart was occluded. The others arteries were normal. We recommended that Al have bypass surgery but they wanted alternatives. We explained that he could live with this artery remaining closed but he could not tolerate any development of atherosclerosis in the other two arteries. Rosemary asked how they could prevent that buildup and the usual instructions of exercise, losing weight and low cholesterol diet were given. Those simple instructions opened up a whole new career for Rosemary which has included the publication of three books and lectures and discussions with university groups, rehabilitation units, church and social groups.

Her first interest was mainly in lowering Al's cholesterol by changes in diet. When Al's ability to prevent the progession of cholesterol buildup in his arteries was shown on repeat angiograms, Rosemary became convinced that she was on the right track. Later when she developed her own osteoporosis, she began to concentrate on dietary means to reverse her low bone density. When her own bone density kept increasing by her change in dietary intake, she became even more enthusiastic. Much later when Al developed a rapidly progressive Alzheimer's syndrome she sought dietary ways to control these three illnesses. Rosemary has done extensive literature research and has been very careful to not be swayed by the publicity of rapidly passing fads. She has accepted information that has only been published in scientific journals or papers by individuals who have done legitimate research in the field of nutrition and/or have appropriate appointments at respected academic institutions. She has spoken with nutritionists throughout the country, she has spoken with nutritionists at several of the major food processing companies and has incorporated all of this information in workable recipes. Rosemary states that the dietary fads and hoaxes that are not beneficial are rather easily identifiable because of their lack of scientific support and the reluctance to have the theories subjected to scientific study.

Rosemary Fisher's greatest contribution has been to incorporate naturally occurring dietary foods, in amounts shown by research for metabolic benefit, into tasteful dietary recipes. She has rejected the urge to add artificial coloring and artificial flavoring to make the meal more palatable. She has used all natural foods, for instance using natural honey as her sweetener. Tremendous amounts of experimentation with different recipes were necessary to get the combination of flavors and consistencies that would make a palatable and enjoyable menu. Al was her major tester and he frequently stated that he certainly tasted some very terrible combinations. Many recipes were abandoned almost instantly but the ones that has survived have proven to be tasty and appealing to many different groups. Rosemary's major proof of palatability is when the grandchildren come back for seconds.

Rosemary Fisher is a very interesting woman in that she started into this quest for incorporating healthy foods into palatable recipes to achieve an appropriate diet for her husband. As she continued to review more and more scientific evaluations of the value of dietary changes, she became convinced of the need for an overall change in the dietary habits of the American population. She has done this by being able to maintain the tastes that we have all become to fond of in prepared and "fast" foods into her new recipes. Demands for her recipes have been met with the publication of several books, this being the most recent and incorporating her research on osteoporosis and Alzheimer's disease. All monies that she has received from her lectures and from her books have been given to charity. She has been particularly interested in the migrant workers in Florida and the Carmelite religious order that cares for the poor in the Philippines and in South America.

Rosemary Fisher is a remarkable woman who has done remarkable research, has published a remarkable book for a remarkable cause. I feel fortunate to have been able to feel her enthusiasm and to share her successes with her.

Robert A. Heinle, M.D.
Clinical Associate Professor of Medicine
University of Rochester
School of Medicine & Dentistry

PREFACE

My way to "Thank God" for giving me good health at age 78 is to share my research findings and recipes with you. Try just one recipe and as you feel better you will be motivated to try more. My recipes are based on research, enabling me to combine the right minerals and vitamins in the right foods in my recipes. This way you can absorb these important minerals and vitamins in the food. If you do not absorb the minerals and vitamins in your food, you will not enjoy the health benefits necessary for good health.

When I first devised the diet in my book, *Osteoporosis, My Story and Diet*, I never thought the diet would benefit those who suffer from osteoporosis, heart disease, cancer and now dementia (Alzheimer's). I am grateful!

At an older age it is wonderful to be able to enjoy independent living. Without good health this would not be possible.

NOTICE

This book is intended as a reference only - not as a medical manual. Your doctor should be consulted about any medical problem. It is not intended to be a substitute for any diet your doctor may have prescribed. To insure good health, your doctor should be consulted for any exercise program you do.

– TABLE OF CONTENTS–

RECITES

RECIPES

MAIN DISHES

VEGETABLES

INTRODUCTION

Each day scientific knowledge grows about the way the foods we eat influence our lives, our health, our activity, and our energy. In the last several years scientists from all over the globe have made substantial strides in proving or disproving the beneficial results of eating different foods. In this book I have tried to assemble summaries of what I consider to be some of the more significant recent research findings and to summarize them in terms that are easy to understand.

I hope you will find in these summaries some useful information that you can apply to your own eating habits. To assist you in this, I have included recipes that I have developed in the second part of the book. The recipes include the vitamins, minerals, and foods mentioned in the research. Each recipe lists the vitamins and minerals that are contained in the recipes so you can select them as needed.

You can also apply the research to your own favorite recipes by noting the principles covered and adjusting your recipes accordingly. Practice the substitutions and enjoy the results.

In changing the foods you eat, remember to take it a step at a time, insuring that the food you prepare is tasty and enjoyable to all who eat it. I hope that the research and recipes in this book will help you to have wonderful tasting food that adds to the quality and energy that you and your loved ones experience in life.

SUMMARY

In the earlier comments made on research findings, I have indicated the source of the information so that you will be encouraged to read the materials and realize that these statements were able to be made because someone did impressive research on the topic. My reason for doing this is because so many people have said to me, "References, I never read them."

Take a step at a time in modifying your diet. Remember though, each step you take is a step toward good health. Best of all, it is a step toward independent living.

The best way to manage osteoporosis, heart disease, cancer, and dementia is to follow a diet to control these diseases. Consult your doctor or health professional regarding a diet and an exercise program suited to you. It is your choice, as it was my choice, to choose to contribute to your own health. My hope is that you will modify your diet and, as you feel better, it will be easier to do more.

In closing, I would like to give my grateful thanks to God for his guidance in enabling me to apply my research findings to my diet, but, most of all, for giving me the ability to develop recipes that can benefit our bones, bodies and minds.

RESEARCH AND RECIPES
ON DEMENTIA, HEART DISEASE
OSTEOPOROSIS & CANCER

RESEARCH

— THIAMINE (VITAMIN B 1) —

OVERVIEW

My interest in thiamine, better known as vitamin B1, started in 1993 when I read a study published in the Annals of Neurology. (Authors Anonymous: Thiamine in Alzheimer's Disease, Annals of Neurology 28 (2): 203-301, 1990.) The study indicated that high doses of thiamine might be beneficial in treating the reduced mental abilities of people afflicted with Alzheimer's disease. I thought to myself, "How great, if, as we age, we could even improve our mental abilities." At that time, I never thought of anyone in our family as having Alzheimer's disease. I was thinking, "What would we have to lose if we were to include foods high in thiamine in our diet? Nothing to lose and everything to gain."

Another study came out later that reinforced the findings of the earlier study. Patients with dementia of Alzheimer type reported significant cognitive improvement with thiamine therapy. (Meador, K.J., Nichols, M.E., Franke, P., Durkin, M.U., Oberzan, R.L., Moore, E.E., Loring, D.W.: Evidence for a Central Cholinergic Effect of High-dose Thiamine in Dementia of Alzheimer's Type Disease; Annals of Neurology 34 (5): 724-726, 1993.) It reconfirmed my interest in increasing our intake of thiamine through foods.

HOW THIAMINE FUNCTIONS

New studies on thiamine are being conducted even today. The range of influence thiamine has on our good health is already impressive. For example, thiamine is essential in the manufacture of hydrochloric acid, thereby helping us absorb our vitamins and minerals. Other functions of thiamine include improving excretion of fluid stored in the body, decreasing rapid heart rate, alleviating fatigue, and improving mental alertness as well as nerve function. Thiamine is known as the "morale vitamin" because of its relation to a healthy nervous system and its beneficial effect on mental attitude.

Thiamine is not stored in the body and therefore must be supplied daily. Because thiamine is excreted in the urine, it is very important that we include thiamine-rich foods in our daily diets. Thiamine is generally excreted at a faster rate during periods of stress. Eating excessive amounts of sugar, as well as smoking and drinking alcohol, will also cause a thiamine depletion.

Researchers also think there may be a link to memory loss, if one's diet is low in vitamin B1 (thiamine). The inability to concentrate may also be associated with a deficiency of thiamine. The study was published in two journals. (Butterworth, R.F., Besard, A.M.: Thiamine-dependent Enzyme Changes in Temporal Cortex of Patient with Alzheimer's Disease, Metal Brain Dis 5: 179-184, 1990 and Nolan, K.A., Black, R.S., Sheu, K.F.R.: Trial of Thiamine in Alzheimer's Type Disease, Archives of Neurology 48: 81-83, 1991.)

THIAMINE AND ANXIETY, DEPRESSION

Researchers have found that even a small deficiency of thiamine, a B1 vitamin, can cause anxiety symptoms. Think how much better our lives could be if we could just reduce our anxiety symptoms.

As early as 1948, researchers were studying the psychological effects of thiamine deficiency on psychiatric patients in an institution. The subjects received varying amounts of thiamine in an adequate diet. They were tested for various deficiency effects. When approximately four tenths of a milligram of thiamine was administered, specific conditions, including loss of inhibitory emotional control, paranoid trends, manic-depressive features, and confusion, were alleviated. (Horwitt, M.K. et al: Investigations of Human Requirements of B-Complex Vitamins, National Research Council Bulletin 116: 1948.)

THIAMINE AND ALHEIMER'S

A study by researcher R.H. Haas in 1988 suggested that a high dose of thiamine helps to restore memory and cognitive function in the early stages of Alzheimer's type dementia patients. (Haas, R.H.: Thiamine and the Brain, Annu Rev Nutr 8: 483-515, 1988.) It is also important to note that at least 40 studies on thiamine and its relationship to Alzheimer's disease have been published since then.

Researcher Meador and colleagues, for example, published two studies showing improvement when high doses of thiamine were administered to Alzheimer's type dementia patients. (Meador, K., Loring, D., Nichols, M., Zanrini, E., Rivner, M., Posas, H., Thompson, E., Moore, E.: Preliminary Findings of High-dose Thiamine in Dementia of Alzheimer's Type, Journal of Geriatrics, Psychiatry, & Neurology 6: 222-229, 1993 and Meador, K.J.,

Nichols, M.E., Franke, P., Durkin, M.U., Oberzan, R.L., Moore, E.E., Loring, D.W.: Evidence for a Central Cholinergic Effect of High-dose Thiamine in Dementia of Alzheimer's Type Disease, Annals of Neurology 34 (5): 724-726, 1993.)

A research publication of June, 1994, stated that University of Florida neurologists at Gainesville are conducting a study on Alzheimer's patients using thiamine. They want to determine whether it can improve memory with fewer side effects than existing medications. They are using supplements in the study to control the amount each person takes.

Use of supplements is great for a study, but if you are trying to increase thiamine in your diet, it is wiser to do it with food. (You will find recipes high in thiamine later in the recipe sections.) In food you can balance the B vitamins and, as a result, they will not compete with each other in the intestines for absorption by the body.

Experiments are still being conducted today on the benefits of including thiamine in our foods. As I noted in the opening, what do we have to lose if we eat thiamine-rich foods? Nothing, and we may just improve our memories and cognitive function. Thiamine may or may not help with Alzheimer's disease, but again, after reading the above research, think of all the health benefits we could gain, using thiamine-rich foods in our daily diets, to help reduce our risk for potential health complications.

– MAGNESIUM –

OVERVIEW

Now let's take a look at the importance of magnesium in our diets. Most of us know the importance of including calcium-rich foods in our diets, but many do not know the importance of including magnesium-rich foods in our diets along with the calcium. Later in this book you will find recipes that will have a good calcium-magnesium ratio, that is, the calcium is closely listed with magnesium as opposed to being separated by other elements.

MAGNESIUM AND CALCIUM

Calcium instructs muscles to contract, magnesium instructs muscles to relax. A high-fat diet can steal both magnesium and calcium. R.B. Singh, M.D., chief cardiologist and professor of clinical nutrition at the Moradabad Medical Hospital in Moradabad, India, discussed this finding. The study suggested that high dietary fat can inhibit the absorption of magnesium, and that we absorb even less magnesium with saturated than with polyunsaturated fat. (Singh, R.B.: A High-fat Diet Can Steal Both Magnesium and Calcium, Journal Magnesium 9: 255, 1990.)

The more calcium in the diet, the more magnesium that is needed. Calcium given alone can induce a magnesium deficiency. The most serious complications from a deficiency of magnesium are heart conditions such as irregular heartbeat and rapid heartbeat. (Bariscoe, M., Ragen, C.: Relation of Magnesium on Calcium Metabolism in Man, American Journal of Nutrition 19: 296, 1966.)

Gustawa Stendig-Lindberg, M.D., of the Sackler School of Medicine at Tel Aviv University, one of the researchers in the study published in the research publication, Medical Tribune, has suggested that, after a woman reaches menopause, bone density usually drops by about one percent a year. It is believed that magnesium may halt the loss of bone because it aids in the transport of calcium in and out of the cells. Magnesium plays an important part in converting vitamin D to its active form. (Stendig-Lindberg, G., M.D.: Medical Tribune: July 22, 1993.) Another good reason to include magnesium in our diet.

MAGNESIUM AND OSTEOPOROSIS

According to Mildred S. Seelig, Ph.D., a magnesium expert from the University of North Carolina, more than half of the body's magnesium is found in the bones. Calcium gives bones their strength, while magnesium helps them maintain their elasticity to prevent injury. (Seelig, M.S.: Increased Magnesium Need with use of Combined Estrogen and Calcium for Osteoporosis, Magnesium Research 3: 197-215, 1990.) This is one good reason to be sure we have a good calcium-magnesium ratio in our daily diet.

In this study on osteoporosis, magnesium and calcium were increased along with estrogen therapy. But, if you are not a candidate for estrogen therapy to prevent (further) osteoporosis, you may want to review the chapter later in this book on SOY (Defatted Soy Flour) to find ways in which defatted soy flour may help you increase the estrogen level in your body through food intake. In my previous books, I also describe foods high in boron that may help increase estrogen levels. (Fisher, R.C.: Osteoporosis, My High Calcium, Low Cholesterol Diet: 12-13, 1989), (Fisher, R.C.: Research and Recipes on Osteoporosis, Heart Disease and Cancer: 7, 1992.) Since I am not a candidate for estrogen therapy, I include these foods in my daily menu.

Guy E. Abraham, M.D., presents data that suggest that magnesium deficiency has a significant role in primary post-menopausal osteoporosis. Magnesium is involved in calcium metabolism and in the synthesis of vitamin D, as well as in maintaining bone integrity. (Abraham, G.E., Grewal, H.: A Total Dietary Program Emphasizing Magnesium Instead of Calcium in the Treatment of Osteoporosis, Journal of Reproductive Medicine 35: 503-507, 1990.) (Abraham, G.E.: The importance of Magnesium in Management of Primary Post-Menopausal Osteoporosis, Journal of Nutritional Medicine 2: 1 65-1 78, 1991.)

A study in Israel found that sixteen out of nineteen women had lower than normal trabecular (hip area) magnesium content and also had lower blood levels of magnesium, as was determined by infrared spectroscopy. (Cohen, L., Kitzes, R.: Infrared Spectroscopy and Magnesium Content of Bone Mineral in Osteoporotic Women, Isr J Med Sci 17: 1123-1125, 1981.)

MAGNESIUM AND THE ELDERLY

The elderly especially need to be aware of a magnesium deficiency. In one case study, a 74 year old woman became confused, slurred her speech and could barely walk. Worried friends rushed the woman to a hospital where doctors discovered her magnesium level was dangerously low. It was discovered the woman was taking calcium supplements, but no magnesium, and eating a nutritionally poor diet. She was treated with magnesium injections and made a complete recovery. (Authors Anonymous: Archives of Internal Medicine 151, 3: 593.) This case study only underscores the importance of a balanced, nutritious diet as well as the importance of avoiding large doses of any supplement without a doctor's supervision.

MAGNESIUM AND HEART

Magnesium is also helpful for people suffering from abnormally rapid heartbeat, known as tachyarrhythmias or tachycardia. Magnesium is safe in reduction of arrhythmias. Magnesium deficiency can be caused by poor diet and some diseases such as gastrointestinal disorders as well as diuretic drugs. (Abraham, A.: Magnesium is Safe in Reduction of Incidence of Arrhythmias, Journal of Magnesium 9: 177, 1990.)

MAGNESIUM AND HEADACHES

A report in the journal Headache suggests that low levels of the mineral magnesium may be closely linked to migraine headaches. (Kahn, J.: Low Ionized Magnesium Linked to Migraine Headaches, Medical Tribune: 7, May 18, 1995.) Even if you do not have a migraine headache, an inexpensive insurance policy would be to eat foods high in magnesium. Note the foods listed in this book that are high in magnesium and include them in your diet. Low magnesium levels may be at least partly to blame for excruciating migraine pain.

MAGNESIUM AND FATIGUE

The association between magnesium status and Chronic Fatigue Syndrome (CFS) was investigated at the University of Southampton, UK. In one study 20 patients with CFS showed lower red blood cell magnesium levels than did healthy people. How magnesium affects CFS is poorly understood. Improvements in energy levels and mood reported in this study correspond with findings of other investigators who used magnesium to treat anxiety, insomnia, and mental disorders. Regardless of the mechanism, patients suffering from chronic fatigue syndrome have low levels of magnesium supplementation. (Cox, I., Campbell, J., Dowson, D.: Red Blood Cell, Magnesium and Chronic Fatigue Syndrome, Lancet 337: 757-760, 1991.)

MAGNESIUM AND DEPRESSION

As long ago as 1973, a Navy physician, Richard Hall reported on a patient suffering from gross deficiency of the mineral magnesium. In the article he listed recognizable symptoms of magnesium deficiency. The symptoms cover many of the psychiatric, neurological and circulatory disorders from which many Americans suffer: depression, marked agitation, disorientation, confusion, irritability, restlessness, muscular weakness, rapid heart beat, high blood pressure, arrhythmia and many more. (Hall, R.: Journal of the American Medical Association: June 25, 1973.) As you can see, there may be many good reasons to increase the magnesium in our diets.

– VITAMIN C –

OVERVIEW

In 1932, researchers identified the unknown substance in lemon juice that prevented scurvy as vitamin C. Vitamin C helps to form and maintain material that holds body cells together and strengthens the walls of blood vessels. It also aids in normal tooth and bone formation, in healing wounds and gives resistance to infections. This chapter will update you on the current research on vitamin C.

VITAMIN C AND LUNG DISEASES

Vitamin C strengthens the lungs, according to a recent study by the Harvard Medical School and the Environmental Agency. Scott Weiss, Ph.D., along with Joel Schwartz, Ph.D., analyzed data from the First National Health and Nutrition Examination Survey. They found that people consuming as little as 178 mg. daily could expel substantially more air from the lungs than those eating only 17 mg. of vitamin C daily. (Schwartz, J.: Vitamin C Important Anti-oxidant that Directly Neutralizes Free Radicals and is Part of Glutathione Peroxidase Pathway for Repairing Oxidative Lipid Membrane, Journal of Clinical Nutrition 59:110-114,1994.) Including vitamin C regularly can be very helpful to those who have breathing difficulties related to some diseases.

A case study on hospital patients with bronchitis and pneumonia, found that these patients recovered faster with a vitamin C supplement. The dose was 200 mg. a day. It is easy to get this amount of vitamin C in our food, if we check the vitamin C content of the food we eat.

VITAMIN C AND CHOLESTEROL

Judith Hallfrisch, Ph.D., of the U.S. Department of Agriculture's Beltsville Human Research Center in Maryland, who studied 827 patients, found some interesting data on vitamin C. Low levels of vitamin C may raise people's total cholesterol level, especially the LDL form of bad cholesterol. However, a modest intake of vitamin C can lower total cholesterol levels and increase the HDL form of good cholesterol.

Hallfrisch also notes that even in a population consuming two to three times the RDA of vitamin C, that less atherogenic (degenerative) profiles can be seen in those with higher plasma concentrations of ascorbic acid or vitamin C. (Hallfrisch, J.: High Plasma Vitamin C Associated with High Plasma HDL and Cholesterol, American Journal of Clinical Nutrition 60:100-5,1994.) By improving cholesterol levels, vitamin C may help reduce the risk of cardiovascular disease.

VITAMIN C AND HEART

Other lab research has suggested that vitamin C may help the heart in other ways. Experimental doses of vitamin C, at 600 mg. a day or more, have made the blood less sticky, which could reduce the risk of heart attack and stroke. Some studies have found that high levels of vitamin C, measured in the blood or in the diet, are associated with lower blood pressure. (Author Anonymous: Can Vitamin C Save Your Life?, Consumer Reports on Health 6: (3) March, 1994.)

VITAMIN C AND AMINO ACIDS

In current research studies on vitamin C by Matthias Rath, M.D., of San Francisco, it was found that amino acids lysine and prolein remove the adhesive quality of fats in the blood so they won't stick to blood vessel walls. This forces the fat deposits from their clogging positions. (Rath, M., M.D.: Today's Breakthroughs: Tomorrow's Cures, Research Summary, Health Now, 387 Ivy Street, San Francisco, CA 94102.)

This study shows the importance of including amino acids in our foods. These amino acids can easily be obtained in appropriate amounts in defatted soy flour. In 3-1/2 ounces of defatted soy flour there are 3300 mg. of lysine and 3040 mg. of prolein. Other sources of amino acids are nuts, yogurt, milk, non-fat dry milk, dairy products, chicken, and turkey.

VITAMIN C AND AGING

A deficiency in vitamin C leads to an older appearance, says Gary S. Ross, M.D., of San Francisco, California, who specializes in preventive medicine. A diet heavy in fresh fruits or 1000 mg. of vitamin C each day aids in forming collagen and gives a smoother appearance. (Orey, C.: Natural Beauty 20 Secrets to Eternal Youth, Let's Live: March, 1994.)

Vitamin C is essential for the formation of collagen, the connective tissue. Therefore, vitamin C helps in the healing of wounds and burns. Vitamin C is also required for maintaining the strength of capillaries. Otherwise we might experience bleeding gums, loosened teeth, and bone fractures. A study in the Academy of General Dentistry reports that vitamin C can assist dental healing after a tooth extraction. (Authors Anonymous: American Journal of Dentistry 5: 269, 1992.) Researchers are not sure how vitamin C helps, but it has long been suspected that vitamin C also plays a role in wound healing.

VITAMIN C AND CANCER

For years when Dr. Linus Pauling noted that ascorbic acid, better known as vitamin C, does more than prevent sniffles, no one seemed to be listening. He said that vitamin C works because it strengthens the immune system and may help to keep tumors from spreading, as it scavenges the body to find and destroy stray cancer cells. (Pauling, L.: Vitamin C Strengthens Immune System and Destroys Cancer Cells, National Cancer Institute Conference, 1993. Linus Pauling Institute of Science and Medicine 440: Page Mill Road, Palo Alto CA 94306.)

Studies noted by Gladys Block, M.D., a National Cancer Institute Epidemiologist at a conference in 1993, however, showed that out of a total of 47 studies, 34 showed that vitamin C had a preventive effect on cancers of the lung, larynx, oral cavity, esophagus, stomach, colon, rectum, pancreas, bladder, brain, endometrium and breast. And its side effects are minimal. (Block, G.: Vitamin C and Cancer, Your Health: July 13,1993.) As I said before, what have we got to lose?

WHEN TO TAKE VITAMIN C

When more than 500 mg. of vitamin C is taken at one time, the body excretes the extra amount of vitamin C. As a result, the least excretion occurs when the vitamin is taken in divided doses three or four times a day (e.g., 500 mg. each time). Also, the greatest absorption from your intake of vitamin C, in a supplement, occurs when you take it after a meal or with food.

If you are taking a vitamin C supplement of more than 1000 mg. per day, remember to include copper-rich foods in your diet. Researchers are saying over 1000 mg. of vitamin C a day in supplemental form could deplete our bodies of copper. Just make sure you include foods rich in copper in your daily diet. Some foods rich in copper are whole grains, legumes, bananas, potatoes, apricots, dates, dried fruits, pecans, broccoli, and grapes.

A precaution. Even 500 mg. of chewable vitamin C can make the mouth acidic enough to start dissolving tooth enamel. The researchers recommend that people buy tablets that can be swallowed. (Authors Anonymous: American Journal of Dentistry 5: 269, 1992.)

GETTING VITAMIN C THROUGH FOOD

When you feel you are coming down with a cold, what is the thing many people do? Increase their intake of vitamin C. Vitamin C (ascorbic acid) is often referred to as the key vitamin in the body. If you take a vitamin C supplement each day, do also try to increase the vitamin C content of your daily foods as well, since foods contain many other vitamins and minerals that supplements will not contain.

Different foods also contain different amounts of vitamin C. Those of us who automatically reach for orange juice as having the highest vitamin C content, for example, will be surprised to realize that an orange and many other fruits and vegetables have a higher content of vitamin C.

Good sources of vitamin C are citrus fruits (oranges, grapefruits, lemons, and their juices), and fresh strawberries. Surprising is the fact that green peppers contain more vitamin C than an orange. Red peppers contain even more vitamin C than green peppers, plus they also contain vitamin A that converts to beta-carotene in the body. Potatoes and sweet potatoes (especially with the skins on), watermelon, and cantaloupes also contain good amounts of vitamin C.

– FOLIC ACID –

OVERVIEW

Many studies are showing the importance of including foods rich in folic acid (folacin or folate) in our diet. For several years increased intake of folic acid has been recommended for pregnant women. Studies have shown it may protect against birth defects. Now more discoveries are showing folic acid may protect against stroke, heart disease and cervical cancer.

FOLIC ACID AND CERVICAL CANCER

According to Charles E. Butterworth, Jr., M.D., and colleagues at University of Alabama in Birmingham, women who have low levels of folic acid, the B vitamin, are more likely to develop early cervical cancer than women with high levels of the vitamin. (Butterworth, C. Jr. et al: Folate Deficiency and Cervical Dysplasia, Journal of American Medical Association 267: 528-533, 1992.)

FOLIC ACID AND HOMOCYSTEINE

Levels of folic acid seem to be related to levels of homocysteine. Homocysteine is an amino acid. Your body produces homocysteine and normally processes it so it is not hazardous to your health. However, sometimes your body cannot process homocysteine quickly enough and then you get a build-up of the amino acid. That's when it can be a problem.

People with too much homocysteine have a higher risk of heart disease. Results: volunteers in a study who had low levels of folic acid or high levels of homocysteine were twice as likely to have arteries that were at least 25 percent clogged. Researchers are not sure that lowering homocysteine levels could prevent heart disease, but, in the meantime, making sure you are getting you are getting at least 400 mcg. of folic acid a day is a good idea. (Salmon, D.P., Thal, L.U., Butters, N., Heidel, W.C.: Low Folic Acid Levels - High Homocysteine Levels May be Risk for Heart Disease, New England Journal of Medicine 332: 286, 1995.)

– SOY (DEFATTED SOY FLOUR) –

OVERVIEW

Many research studies are showing us the importance of including soy foods in our daily diet. I am finding that defatted soy flour is being used by many researchers in their research studies. A good example is a study by Mark Wahlqvist, professor of medicine at Monash University in Victoria, Australia. He and his team studied the effect of three foods reported to induce vaginal oestrus (estrogen) in laboratory animals, and used the results in a study of post menopausal women not taking estrogen replacement therapy.

SOY AND ESTROGEN

According to Wahlqvist, a sensitive indicator of estrogenic activity is vaginal cell maturation. Vaginal smears revealed significantly increased estrogenic activity in the women eating the soy flour. To increase their estrogen levels as they did, they had eaten about 3-1/2 tablespoons of defatted soy flour a day in their diets. The 25 postmenopausal women in the study ranged in age from 51 to 70 years. (Wahlqvist, M.L., FRACP: Soy Mimics Female Hormone Estrogen, British Medical Journal 301: 905-6, 1990.)

When I saw this study, I was impressed. I personally am not a candidate for estrogen replacement therapy, so I was thrilled to find something in research studies on food that could perhaps help me. Phytoestrogens are found in only some plants and mimic the female hormone estrogen. Soybeans are plants that contain the phytoestrogens, and soy flour is a derivative of the soybean.

Dr. Herman Aldercreutz of the University of Helsinki in Finland reported that for those beyond the reproducing years, phytoestrogens can be highly beneficial. (Aldercreutz, H., Fotsis, T., Bannwart, C., Brunow, C., Hose, T.A.: Isotope Dilution Gas Chromatographic-mass Spectrometric Method of the Determination of Lignans and Isoflavonoids in Human Urine, Including Identification of Genistein, Chin Chim Acta 199: 263-278, 1991.) As an example, a diet moderately high in phytoestrogens over a lifetime, especially in women whose estrogen production has virtually stopped, may diminish a person's risk for late onset of chronic diseases.

Dr. Aldercreutz has been one of the most productive researchers in the field of phytoestrogens in plants for the past 20 years. I personally have copies of at least 10 of his studies that have been published in various journals.

SOY AND CANCER

Dr. Aldercreutz also suggests a link between the typical Western diet, which is low in phytoestrogens, and the development of hormone-dependent cancers such as breast, prostate, endometrial, ovarian, colon, as well as heart disease. (Aldercreutz, H., Fotsis, T., Bannwart, C., Wahala: Determination of Urinary Lignans and Phytoestrogen Metabolites, Potential Antiestrogen and Anticarcinogens in Urine of Women on Various Habitual Diets, Steroid Biochem 25: 791-797, 1986.)

SOY AND TAMOXIFEN

In some studies scientists report finding tamoxifen-like substances in soybeans that may block tiny "seeds" of estrogen-dependent breast cancer early in the disease process, before estrogen receptors have had a chance to go bad.

Stephen Barnes, a pharmacologist at the University of Alabama at Birmingham, and his colleagues reported results on rats, suggesting that a tamoxifen look-alike found in soybeans may block cancer at an early stage, presumably when the estrogen receptors still function. They say their findings may help explain why Japanese and Chinese women who eat lots of soy-rich foods have a much lower incidence of breast cancer than women in the United States.

Rats eating the most soy had the fewest breast tumors. Barnes tentatively attributes these results to a compound called genistein, which is found in soybeans and which resembles estrogen and tamoxifen in structure. Like tamoxifen, genistein may discourage tumor growth by blocking estrogen receptors, he speculates. (Barnes, S. et al: Soy Creates Compound Genistein, Science News 137: 19, 1994.)

In the University of Texas Lifetime Health Letter, September 1994, it was reported that Dr. Barnes and his colleagues are studying a group of phytochemicals known as isoflavones, which are chemically similar to estrogen. In an ongoing clinical study, the investigators hope to identify certain blood and tissue proteins that may serve as cancer markers ("red flags" that may signal cancer). Then they will evaluate the effects of the soy extracts on the markers.

SOY AND OSTEOPOROSIS

Although most of the attention has centered on soy's role in reducing cancer and heart disease risks, Dr. Barnes also believes soy products may have great potential in the prevention or treatment of osteoporosis.

Because these soy phytonutrients are estrogen-normalizing, it has also been proposed that in menopausal women they may have a beneficial effect in preventing bone loss due to osteoporosis (associated with the loss of estrogen production by the ovaries). Soy protein was used in this study that found that vitamins and amino acids are helpful for calcium absorption. (Barnes, S. et al: Soy Creates Compound Genistein, Science News 137: 19, 1994.) Research is also showing that when we shift from a diet high in red meat to a diet high in soy (plant-foods), we excrete less calcium in our urine, thus helping to decrease our risk of osteoporosis.

Researchers Vernon Young, Ph.D., and Nevin Scrimshaw, Ph.D., at the Massachusetts Institute of Technology at Cambridge, have found the protein produced in the soybean is such high quality, it is capable of supporting the body's need for essential amino acids. (Young, V., Scrimshaw, S.: Soybean Protein is Capable of Supporting Body's Need for Amino Acids, American Journal of Clinical Nutrition 59: SS, 12035-12125,1994.)

An additional explanation about soy foods in our diets. Phytoestrogens called isoflavone phytoestrogens are modified in the colon by bacteria and absorbed into the body where they have estrogen or anti-estrogen activities in different tissues. Watch for more news on these phytochemicals in the media. Many of the phytochemicals may become part of our diets, as we realize their importance for us in maintaining our good health.

SOY AND CHOLESTEROL

According to Dr. James Anderson and colleagues at the University of Alabama, soy protein may reduce your blood-fat levels. (Anderson, J.W., Johnstone, B.M., Cook-Newell, M.E.: Meta-analysis Effects of Soy Protein Intake on Serum Lipids, New England Journal of Medicine 333: 276-286, 1995.) The investigators reviewed 38 clinical trials in which dietary protein from meat was replaced with soy protein. They found that people who ate soy protein had a 9 percent greater reduction in total cholesterol than people who ate meat. Reductions were 13 percent greater in the LDL (bad cholesterol) and 11 percent in the triglycerides in people on the soy diet compared to those who ate meat. Triglycerides are now being recognized as a blood fat involved in heart disease.

Dr. Carroll also reviewed clinical studies on soy protein lowering cholesterol. He found a significant decrease in plasma total and LDL cholesterol on a diet high in soy protein. (Carroll, K.K.: Review of Clinical Studies on Cholesterol-lowering Response to Soy Protein, Am Diet Assoc 9: 820-827, 1991.)

SOY AND MINERALS

Soy is a great example of a food that contains a good number of minerals. The availability of calcium in soybeans is almost as good as that in milk. Defatted soy flour is one of the highest sources of protein, potassium, magnesium, calcium, and thiamine. It is also the lowest in fat of all the soy products, as well as the highest in protein (folic acid, another B vitamin, that is needed to metabolize protein). I find it very easy to add soy to my recipes in the form of defatted soy flour, one of the highest sources of soy protein. I hope this is encouragement for you to try my recipes that include defatted soy flour.

SOY AND ALZHEIMER'S

Researchers who study Alzheimer's disease have found nerve cells require acetylcholine to send impulses. In what is known as Alzheimer's disease and in subsequent senile dementia, activity of choline acetyltansferase has been found, according to Abram Hoffer, M.D. (Hoffer, A., M.D., Ph.D.: Orthomolecular Medicine for Physicians, New Canaan, Conn.: Keats Publishing, Inc., 1989.)

In a study at National Institute of Mental Health when patients were given choline there was some improvement in memory, more pronounced in the subjects who were the worst. (Murray, F.: Alzheimer's Treatment & Causes, Better Nutrition: 11, May, 1990.)

Another good reason to include soy flour in our diets. A large percentage of the choline circulating in blood plasma comes from eating foods containing lecithin. Lecithin supplements are usually derived from soybeans. Soy flour is a derivative of the soybean as well, and contains both choline and lecithin. Defatted soy flour gives us the soy without the fat.

− PHYTOSTEROLS −

OVERVIEW

We discussed phytoestrogens, now what about phytosterols? According to Claude L. Hughes Jr., M.D., Ph.D., of Duke University, Durham, NC, phytosterols are present in plants and alter the metabolism of human cholesterol. Though these hormone-like compounds found in edible plants may inhibit a woman's fertility, they may increase her resistance to such chronic diseases as breast and ovarian cancer. People who consume high levels of foods that contain phytosterols also have low risks of developing colon cancer. These people excrete more body generated cholesterol and dietary cholesterol making them less likely to be converted to cancer-causing byproducts in the digestive tract.

Dr. Hughes' studies are described in more detail in his chapter, "Plant Sterols", in the book Infertility and Reproductive Medicine Clinics of North America. The book contains a collection of essays by international experts assembled by the National Center of Toxicologic Research in Jefferson County, Arkansas. (Murray, F.: Compounds Found in Edible Plants May Increase Resistance to Breast and Ovarian Cancer, Better Nutrition: 18, November 18, 1992.)

FOODS RICH IN PHYTOSTEROLS

Remember you must cut the fat and LDL cholesterol in your diet. To do so, increase the whole grains and make sure you include phytosterol-rich foods in your daily diet. After oils, which we ought to limit in our diets, rice bran has the highest amount of phytosterols, almost as high as the corn and wheat germ oils. The next highest food source, but much lower than rice bran, is soybeans. Other foods that contain phytosterols are almonds, peas, and kidney beans. Recipes including these foods are presented in the following chapters.

– BETA-CAROTENE –

OVERVIEW

For years we never thought of foods high in beta-carotene as being effective against diseases, but impressive studies are showing us how important it is to include foods high in beta-carotene in our daily diet. Remember, these studies are with foods high in beta-carotene and not beta-carotene supplements. The fruits and vegetables in which beta-carotene and other members of the carotenoid family can be found also offer other important nutrients, such as vitamins, minerals, and fiber.

BETA-CAROTENE AND ALZHEIMER'S

Blood levels of the vitamins and carotenoids (beta-carotene) are low in Alzheimer's patients, possibly exposing brain neurons to increased oxidative damage. Alzheimer's patients had low vitamin E and beta-carotene levels as compared to healthy individuals. (Zaman, Z., Roche, S., Fielder, P. et al: Plasma Concentrations of Vitamin A and E Carotenoids in Alzheimer's Disease, Age & Aging 21: 91-94, 1992.)

BETA-CAROTENE AND CANCER

Susan Taylor Mayne, Ph.D., and colleagues have pointed out that lung cancer in nonsmokers is responsible for more deaths than cancer of the oral cavity and pharynx, larynx, esophagus, stomach, bone, testis or bladder, multiple myeloma or Hodgkin's disease. (Mayne, S.T., Ph.D. et al: Lung cancer in nonsmokers, Journal of the National Cancer Institute: January 5, 1994.) Previous studies, as well as this study, have shown that eating fruits and vegetables rich in beta-carotene did provide some protection to smokers. Next, the research team wants to see if the same protection can reduce the risk in nonsmoking men and women.

PROTECTIVE BETA-CAROTENE IN
FRUITS AND VEGETABLES

Fruits and vegetables high in beta-carotene, especially when eaten raw, are associated with a reduced risk of lung cancer. There are exceptions, as research is now showing that carrots especially release more carotene, both alpha- and beta-carotene, when they are lightly cooked, but not mushy. According to research conducted by the University of Illinois, heat releases beta-carotene and protein better than chewing does. The best method for cooking is microwaving. Next best is stir-frying (make sure to use only a small amount of oil when stir-frying) followed by quick-steaming. (Authors Anonymous, University of Illinois: Heat Releases Beta-Carotene and Protein Better than Chewing Does, METLIFE, Health Beat Bulletin 2 (1): January, 1995.)

In reviewing 156 studies of fruit and vegetable intake and cancer risk, Gladys Block, Ph.D., professor of public health at the University of California at Berkeley, found that 128 of these studies supported the protective effect of beta-carotene rich foods. (Block, G. et al.: Fruits, Vegetables and Cancer Prevention, A Review of the Epidemiological Evidence, Nutrition and Cancer 18(1): September, 1992.)

This was the most consistent relationship between diet and cancer they had found. In the Nutrition and Cancer article, Dr. Block analyzed the numerous studies that investigated the relationship of beta-carotene and other nutrients to cancer. Seventeen case-control studies of the role of diet in lung cancer were conducted in six countries and all suggested a protective effect of frequent fruit and/or vegetable consumption.

While it may seem difficult to consume five servings of fruits and vegetables daily, Dr. Block suggested that we eat at least one vegetable with our meals and some fruit as a snack. People who eat more fruits and vegetables, especially those rich in the carotenes, usually have a lower risk of most cancers.

To date studies have been reported on the influence of carotenoids in foods. The studies seem to demonstrate that people who eat more foods rich in beta-carotene have a lower risk of cancer. On the other hand, the studies haven't shown that taking beta-carotene supplements lowers cancer risk.

BETA-CAROTENE AND PROSTATE CANCER

In a large-scale study, researchers report that a lower blood vitamin A level increases the likelihood of developing prostate cancer. Men with the lowest vitamin A levels have twice the risk as those with the highest levels of vitamin A. This study provides evidence that a relationship exists between low levels of vitamin A and prostate cancer. (Reichman, M., Hayes et al: Vitamin A and Subsequent Development of Prostate Cancer, First National Health and Nutrition Examination Survey, Epidemiologic Follow-Up Study, Cancer Research 50: 2311-2315, 1990.)

BETA-CAROTENE AND VISUAL DEGENERATION

A recent report has linked daily consumption of fruits and vegetables rich in vitamin A - like carrots, sweet potatoes, pumpkin, brussel sprouts, and squash - to a lower risk of developing macular degeneration. This condition is one of the leading causes of irreversible blindness in people over the age of 65. (Bruce, G.E.: Nutrition and Eye Disease of the Elderly, Journal of Nutritional Biochemistry 5: 66-76,1994.)

Dozens of studies have now shown that beta-carotene, which the body converts into vitamin A, may inhibit the development of cancer and cataracts, as well as strengthening the immune system. Researchers are continuing to build up evidence that cataracts might be preventable.

In a study by the United States Department of Agriculture, scientists discovered that people who ate less than one and a half servings a day of vitamin-rich fruits and vegetables were three and a half times more likely to develop cataracts than people who ate more. In other words, vitamin-rich fruits and vegetables may help you ward off the "inevitable" development of cataracts. More research is needed before anyone can promise you a cataract preventive. In the meantime, however, it won't hurt to get these vitamins in your diet.

Eat fruits and vegetables that are high in vitamin A. Most clinicians advise that we get these nutrients from food, because most studies have examined antioxidants in foods rather than supplements. We know that vegetables high in beta-carotene, for example, protect us, but we don't yet know if their protection comes from beta-carotene or another carotenoid in the same food. More research is being done every day.

In foods there are a variety of carotenoids that benefit our bodies in many ways. You can see a number of these in Table 1. The last three carotenoids are not usually found in supplements.

TABLE 1

WHERE TO GET WHICH CAROTENOIDS

Alpha-Carotene   canned pumpkin, carrots

Beta-Carotene   canned pumpkin,
                             sweet potatoes, carrots,
                             apricots, spinach,
                             collard greens,
                             cantaloupe

Beta-Cryptoxanthin   papaya, oranges,
                             tangerines

Lutein and Zeaxanthin   kale, collard greens,
                             swiss chard,
                             mustard greens,
                             red pepper, okra,
                             romaine lettuce

Lycopene   tomato juice,
                             watermelon,
                             guava,
                             pink grapefruit,
                             tomatoes

(Authors Anonymous: Nutrition Action Healthletter, January and February 1995.)

ALPHA-CAROTENE VS. BETA-CAROTENE

In a laboratory study reported in the Journal of the National Cancer Institute, Japanese researchers reported that alpha-carotene was 10 times more effective in reducing tumor growth than beta-carotene. (Authors Anonymous: Alpha-carotene Versus Beta-carotene, Journal National Cancer Institute 81, 21:1649,1990.)

After reading about all these research studies, I think you'll agree with me that if we want to benefit our bodies, it is wise to eat a variety of fruits and vegetables that are high in beta-carotene and all the carotenoids - vitamin A. This way we are sure to obtain some of the benefits noted in the research studies.

Table II suggests the percent of RDA (Recommended Daily Allowance) for a number of foods that contain a higher amount of Vitamin A. Some other foods that have a high content of total carotenoids are tomato juice canned, dried apricots, watermelon, pink grapefruit, romaine lettuce, celery, and endive lettuce.

TABLE II

ANTIOXIDANT VITAMIN A CONTENT
OF SELECTED FRUITS AND VEGETABLES

Food	Service Size %	Vitamin A % Percentage U.S. RDA
Pumpkin, canned	1 cup	540
Carrots	1 cup	384
Sweet potato, peeled	1 cup	249
Butternut squash	1 cup	175
Spinach, cooked	1 cup	172
Spinach, raw	1 cup	45
Swiss chard	1 cup	120
Kale	1 cup	96
Mango, sliced	1 cup	64
Sweet red peppers	1 cup	58
Cantaloupe	1 cup	52
Mandarin oranges, canned	1 cup	21
Asparagus	1 cup	16
Tomato	medium	14

(Authors Anonymous: ESHA Research, Salem Oregon,
Nutrition Action Healthletter: Jan./Feb. 1995.)

– CALCIUM –

OVERVIEW

It is important for you to know that 99% of the calcium we ingest is incorporated into our bones and teeth. Think about what the remaining 1% has to do in our bodies. It is important in nerve transmission, muscle contraction and relaxation, blood clotting and membrane permeability, to just naming a few of its functions.

When I met Dr. Donald Chan, a Professor at University of Rochester Medical School, he gave me some words of wisdom. "It is not just important to ingest the calcium, but it is important how much you absorb of the calcium you take in." His words really made me stop and think. I decided to find out all about the bone-robbers, foods that rob the bones of calcium, and try to reduce them in my daily diet so I could better absorb my calcium.

It is also important to include other foods high in minerals and vitamins that help us to absorb calcium and thereby help our bodies. I have explained this in detail in one of my other books. (Fisher, R.C.: Osteoporosis: My High Calcium, Low Cholesterol Diet: 2-4, 9-15, 1989.)

NON-FAT DRY MILK AND CALCIUM

I also add non-fat dry milk to my yogurt recipe, in a fairly large amount, to increase the vitamin D as well as the magnesium content in the recipe. Generally, store bought yogurt is not known to have a really high vitamin D content. When you make your own yogurt, and my recipe is so simple, you can be sure you have a good concentration of the minerals and vitamins in it (as opposed to having sugar and fat content). It also has the live cultures so important in absorbing the vitamins and minerals.

INCREASING ABILITY TO ABSORB CALCIUM

As we age, we have a decrease of hydrochloric acid secretion in our bodies and therefore our ability to absorb our calcium declines. Yogurt, being an acid, helps to stimulate the hydrochloric secretion and thereby we are helped to absorb our calcium better. People who eat calcium-rich foods have a lower risk of kidney stones than those who take supplements. (Reid, I., Ames, R., Evans, M., Gamble, D., Sharpe, S.: Increasing Ability to Absorb Calcium, New England Journal of Medicine 328: 833, 1993.)

When buying orange juice I buy the calcium fortified orange juice. I need all the help I can get. I also buy the calcium enriched wheat bread. I find this helpful if I am in a hurry or if I am traveling.

– YOGURT –

OVERVIEW

Though yogurt can be a significant factor in maintaining or increasing our body levels of calcium, it provides many other benefits as well. It helps fight disease and increases our immune system defenses.

YOGURT AND THE IMMUNE SYSTEM

Researchers at the University of California at Davis School of Medicine have found a link between eating yogurt and a healthy immune system. The subjects who ate the yogurt with the live cultures produced four times more gamma interferon, one of the immune system's defenses, than people in the other groups. The group ate 2 cups of yogurt with the live culture daily. (Authors Anonymous, University of California at Davis School of Medicine: Calcium, Vitamins and Other Minerals in Yogurt, International Journal of Immunotherapy 7: 205-210, 1992.) This study may not prove that eating yogurt will guarantee that your immune system will fight off any disease, but finding a way to strengthen your defense against any disease certainly is a good reason to add yogurt to your daily diet. Your body will also benefit from the calcium and other minerals as well as the vitamins in the yogurt.

YOGURT AND LACTOSE INTOLERANCE

As people get older, they usually have a common problem, lactose intolerance. It is the inability to digest lactose, which is found in milk and some other dairy products. At this time about 75% of older adults have lactose intolerance. The symptoms of lactose intolerance include bloating, abdominal cramps, and diarrhea after eating or drinking dairy products.

Instead of eating the offending dairy products, eat yogurt. Even if you have lactose intolerance, you can usually tolerate yogurt. It is low in lactose. Live, active-culture yogurt is the best tolerated. The active cultures in yogurt allow lactose-intolerant people to digest the yogurt and not have the problems associated with lactose intolerance. If you make your own yogurt, you can be sure it has the live active culture.

GETTING MORE MAGNESIUM INTO YOGURT

In the recipe section I have included an easy recipe for making yogurt. When you make it, the yogurt will not only contain live active cultures, but will also have a high calcium and magnesium content. Milk and milk products are very low in magnesium, but with the addition of the dry milk in my recipe you will increase the magnesium content as well as the calcium content. Research is showing that we should have almost as much magnesium as calcium in a recipe to benefit our bodies and our bones.

YOGURT AND VITAMIN K

We should also note that yogurt is a source of vitamin K. By including yogurt in your diet the body may be able to manufacture sufficient amounts of vitamin K. Vitamin K forms a chemical that is required for blood clotting. It is required for a healthy immune system and for normal liver function. It is also thought to play a part in vitality and longevity.

YOGURT AND VAGINAL INFECTIONS

According to Eileen Hilton, M.D., who conducted a study at Long Island Medical Center, women with candidal vaginitis improved dramatically after eating one cup of yogurt daily. (Hilton, E.: Yogurt can be an Effective Treatment for Vaginal C. Albicans Infections, Annals of Internal Medicine 116: 353-357, 1992.)

A French study revealed yogurt not only knocks out yeast infections, it does a one-two punch on cataracts, too. Researchers aren't sure how this works, but it seems that people who eat the most yogurt are the least likely to develop cataracts. (Author Anonymous: Weight Loss and Yogurt Keep You Clear of Cataracts, Natural Healing Newsletter 8 (89): 8, 1996.)

This is one of the many benefits you obtain from eating your cup of yogurt each day. Try my easy recipe for making your own yogurt (recipe section under YOGURT). By making yogurt from this recipe, you will not only have a higher magnesium content, but a higher calcium content as well.

– POTASSIUM –

OVERVIEW

Potassium is a vital mineral and plays an important role in keeping our bodies in "top" condition. Important in helping your body's nervous system to function normally, potassium works closely with other minerals. It works with magnesium in the metabolism of amino acids and helps calcium utilize the carbohydrates. It also helps calcium in the maintenance of nerves.

Homemade yogurt is a very good source of calcium, magnesium and potassium. Since potassium is a very important mineral, we should also include food high in potassium in our daily foods.

SYMPTOMS OF POTASSIUM DEFICIENCY

Potassium deficiency is a common problem in the elderly. Many of the symptoms of potassium deficiency could be depression, fatigue, sleeplessness, muscle weakness and nervousness.

What does all this tell us? Simply, eat a balanced diet that includes the important minerals and vitamins to enjoy better health. Also work at eliminating or reducing the robbers of potassium in our bodies.

HOW YOU MAY BE DEPLETING
YOUR BODY OF POTASSIUM

Sodium may be depleting your body of potassium, as well as calcium. As Adele Davis has explained in one of her many books, sodium exists just outside the cell wall. The sodium may have originally come from meat or table salt. In some way, sodium carries on a lifelong duel with potassium, largely in the cell. When sodium seems to dominate, the cell contains more water, but potassium is withdrawn and excreted in the urine. When potassium is dominant, much sodium and water are lost. (Seelig, M.S.: The Requirement of Magnesium by the Normal Adult, American Journal of Clinical Nutrition XIV: 342, 1964.)

Good reason to reduce our intake of sodium. Eating potassium and magnesium rich foods will usually help the problem, since too little magnesium can also lower potassium absorption.

POTASSIUM AND HEART

Richard Passwater, Ph.D. has suggested that because magnesium is involved in the retention of potassium in the cells, a deficiency of magnesium results in a deficiency of potassium, which may be even worse than a magnesium deficiency in terms of resulting heart damage. This deficiency produces an electrolyte imbalance directly responsible for arrythymia, heart failure, and cell death, as well as death to the individual. (Murray, F.: The Ups and Downs of Potassium Levels, Better Nutrition: 23, November 1989.)

Diuretics (drugs usually given to control high blood pressure) may also reduce your potassium levels. Check with your doctor, if you are taking a diuretic, to see if your drug will reduce your potassium level. Your doctor may want you to include more potassium-rich foods in your diet.

– VITAMINS AND MINERALS –

OVERVIEW

As you can probably guess by now, getting a good combination of vitamins and minerals in our daily food, is an easy way to ensure a healthier life style. Tables lll and IV list some of the easily available foods that we can incorporate into our meals.

TABLE III	
FOOD SOURCES OF SELECTED VITAMINS	
Biotin	brewers yeast, defatted soy flour, whole grains, wheat germ, rice bran, oatmeal, lentils, non-fat yogurt, skim milk, non-fat dry milk, dairy products, chick peas, kidney beans, legumes
Choline	brewers yeast, defatted soy flour, soybeans, wheat germ
Folic Acid	green leafy vegetables such as brussel sprouts, spinach, dark green lettuce, in many fruits, including apples and oranges, yogurt, milk and milk products, fish, eggs, and tuna fish
Niacin	brewers yeast, non-fat dry milk, defatted soy flour, dairy products, breast of turkey, breast of chicken, fish, green vegetables
Vitamin B1 *(thiamine)*	brewers yeast, rice bran, defatted soy flour, wheat germ, oatmeal
Vitamin B12 *(cobalamin)*	brewers yeast, oysters, non-fat yogurt, milk, dairy products, cottage cheese, eggs, turkey, chicken, tuna
Vitamin B2 *(riboflavin)*	brewers yeast, non-fat yogurt, skim milk, non-fat dry milk, dairy products, defatted soy flour, whole grains

Continued on following page

Continued from previous page

Vitamin B6 *(pyridozine)*	brewers yeast, bananas, rice bran, defatted soy flour, whole grains, wheat germ, yogurt, dairy products, oatmeal, brown rice, turkey, chicken, salmon steak, halibut, tuna, nuts, brown rice, green leafy vegetables
Vitamin C	oranges, orange juice, citrus fruits, cantaloupe, tomatoes, green and red peppers, papaya, strawberries, broccoli
Vitamin D	sunlight (not if you are using sunscreen) milk, yogurt, dairy products, non-fat dry milk, fish, mainly sardines, salmon, herring, mackerel, tuna
Vitamin E	wheat germ, rice bran, whole grains, oatmeal, nuts, eggs, legumes, green leafy vegetables
Vitamin K	broccoli, lettuce, cabbage, spinach, yogurt
Vitamin P *(bioflavonoids)*	fruits (skins and pulp), apricots, cherries, grapes, white segment of oranges and grapefruit

TABLE IV

FOOD SOURCES OF SELECTED MINERALS

Calcium	yogurt, skim milk (skim milk is higher in calcium than whole milk), non-fat dry milk, defatted soy flour and soy products, dark green vegetables
Chromium	brewers yeast, wheat germ, prunes, whole grains, rice bran, defatted soy flour, peas, peanut butter, broccoli
Copper	whole grains, rice bran, defatted soy flour, wheat germ, raisins, nuts, legumes, seafood, green leafy vegetables, peas
Iron	brewers yeast, defatted soy flour, rice bran, whole grains, clams, peas, dried apricots, raisins, turkey
Magnesium	rice bran, defatted soy flour, toasted wheat germ, whole grains, beans, non-fat dry milk, brown rice, peanut butter, walnuts and other nuts, oats (lightly cooked, I cook mine in the micro-wave oven), fresh corn, chick peas, eggs
Manganese	rice bran, defatted soy flour, whole grains, oatmeal, pineapple, green vegetables
Potassium	wheat germ, rice bran, defatted soy flour, bananas, dates, raisins, apricots, potatoes (especially with the skins on), oatmeal, non-fat dry milk, winter squash, nuts, skim milk, chicken, turkey, rainbow trout, cod, trout, canned tuna fish
Zinc	rice bran, defatted soy flour, whole grains, wheat germ, mushrooms, seafood especially oysters, nuts, yogurt, milk, dairy products

VITAMINS AND MINERALS SUMMARY

I try to include foods high in the B vitamins in my recipes. They are all needed for our good health, but minerals and trace minerals are also needed. A good example is manganese. It is needed for the metabolism of vitamin B1 and the utilization of vitamin E.

Vitamin A is needed for body tissue repair and maintenance (to resist infection). Magnesium is needed for the metabolism of calcium and vitamin C. One of the most important reasons for having a diet high in the B vitamins is that we eat so many foods that are processed, and processed foods often have had the B vitamins removed. These are just a few examples of the importance of including foods high in vitamins and minerals in our diets.

– ADDITIONAL IDEAS –

TASTY ALTERNATIVES TO SUGAR

It is impossible to pick up a newspaper or magazine without reading how refined sugars are bad for your health. But how much is too much? And what are the alternatives?

The types of sugars that concern nutritionists are the simple processed sugars that have been added to foods. The U.S. Senate Committee that formulated U.S. dietary goals in 1987 estimated that Americans consume about 24% of their calories from sugar. Almost all simple sugars have the same number of calories, about 4 per gram or 155 per ounce.

WHY REDUCING SUGARS IS NECESSARY

These simple sugars occupy an increasing portion of the calories we consume, but they are just about devoid of any nutrients. When we ingest sugar, our bodies take what is needed from the sugar for glucose and the rest of the sugar is converted to fat in the body with potential to clog the arteries (tryglicerides). The more extra sugar we eat, the more we are adding to our fat storage. That's why sugar is so often called "empty calories".

We get sugar in so many foods (check the ingredients on the nutrition label of the foods bought) that we probably have more than enough to satisfy our body system. Refined sugars and processed foods are not only low in nutrients but can also be high in additional fat. In addition, researchers have found that foods containing refined sugar can actually make you hungrier, which can also lead to weight gain.

When we increase our intake of sugars, we are decreasing our consumption of fresh fruits and vegetables, as well as complex carbohydrates that contain important minerals, vitamins and fiber. Not only are we not consuming necessary nutrients, but we are promoting tooth decay with our high consumption of refined sugars.

U.S. dietary goals suggest that refined sugars should comprise not more than 10% of the total calories we eat a day. That means 200 calories for a person who eats 2000 calories a day. There are so many foods containing sugar that it is difficult to estimate exactly how much we eat. It is best to simply limit our intake.

SUBSTITUTES FOR REFINED SUGARS

As a result of our learnings, we should probably work to lower our intake of sugar overall. We may be surprised by the number of new tastes we will discover. But, if we need sugar or crave sweetness, a good source that provides many other benefits is fresh fruit - of any kind. Substituting fresh fruits for sugar will also make you feel fuller, helping you to eat less.

Tupelo honey is another good substitute for refined sugars in recipes. It is a nutritious way to satisfy that sugar craving. I use Tupelo honey, because it is the one type of honey that has the greatest amount of levulose (fructose). Levulose occurs naturally in honey as fructose does in fruits. It is available in most health stores. Remember though, that Tupelo honey has to be used in moderation. It is not a substitute for unlimited use of sugar. A smaller amount of honey can be used in recipes since it is so sweet. Recipes using Tupelo honey are included in the recipe section of this book.

Raisins are a particularly good source for filling recipes or our craving for sweets. They are not low in calories, since there are 240 calories in a 1/2 cup, but they are stuffed with nutrition, including iron and potassium. They are low in sodium, high in fiber and 98% fat free.

DIETARY HABITS: A SIGNIFICANT IMPACT ON HEALTH

Simple changes in your eating habits can decrease your chances of getting some diseases and in some cases even reverse the effects of the disease. Numerous studies have shown that a diet low in fat and high in fiber, can offer protection against some kinds of cancer and may help lower cholesterol. It may also be helpful in the control of diabetes. Perhaps some day we will find that diseases we had attributed to genetic causes may have been due to generations of eating the wrong kinds of foods, or not enough of the right foods.

HIGH FIBER DIETS AND HEALTH

Cultures that have high fiber diets have lower incidence of some kinds of cancer. The average American only consumes about 10-20 grams of fiber daily, which is about half of the 25-35 grams of fiber the National Cancer Institute recommends.

Why fiber protects the body against some diseases isn't known. One reason may be that fiber speeds up the transit time of food through the intestines which may, in case of cancer, minimize the effect of cancer causing agents.

TYPES OF FIBER

It is important to realize that there are two kinds of fiber. First, there is insoluble fiber that does not dissolve in water. It speeds up the digestion process acting like a laxative. Some sources of insoluble fiber are the whole grains, like wheat, rye and bran.

Second, there is soluble fiber that dissolves in water. It slows the stomach's digestive process.

Some sources are vegetables, such as potatoes, carrots, peas, and beans, fruit (all types), and oats. Soluble fiber is thought to help decrease the amount of cholesterol circulating in your blood and may also help control your blood sugar level.

As you can see, it is important to eat a wide variety of fibrous foods, since there are different kinds of fiber. You should be sure to drink a lot of liquids, otherwise fibers can be constipating instead of stimulating.

Whenever I am asked how I was able to change my dietary habits of a lifetime I respond, "It was really common sense, it wasn't easy." I had a sweet tooth, and it was difficult to cut out sweets totally. However, I learned to modify my recipes, so I could still enjoy the food that I was eating.

BENEFITS OF OATMEAL

Oatmeal was mentioned in historical documents as far back as the Bronze Age. The Scots are thought to be the first to recognize the value of oats as food for humans. Early Scots ground oats between stones, then mixed this crude meal with water or other liquid and baked the mixture into thick oat cakes. Oatmeal was first introduced into the USA. about the year 1854.

As children, many of us were sent off to school with hot oatmeal for breakfast. Today oatmeal has been increasingly replaced with many of the boxed cereals that are high in refined sugar, even though researchers are saying loud and clear that oatmeal is good for you.

Oatmeal, when combined with a low fat diet, has been shown to lower cholesterol. Oatmeal is also one of the best sources of soluble fiber. Soluble fiber dissolves in water and slows down your stomach's digestion process. On the glycemic level for a diabetic diet, it is a cereal that would raise blood sugar the least.

Oats are high in protein and do not contain salt or sugar. They contain nine of the eleven B vitamins. They are especially high in vitamin B1 (thiamine). I cook my oatmeal in the microwave oven for just one minute to preserve the high level of thiamine in the oatmeal. Oatmeal also contains vitamin E, magnesium, potassium, phosphorous, iron, zinc, copper and calcium.

Oat products carry more of the original oat kernel than do most other processed cereals. For this reason they lose fewer nutrients between the field and your table. I have a bowl of oatmeal every day for breakfast. I never liked oatmeal as a child, but when I found out how good it was for overall health, I learned to like it as an adult.

ADDITIONAL HINTS

A good reason for drinking skim milk is the recent data that one cup of whole milk has 8 grams of total fat and 5 grams of saturated fat, while 2 percent milk had 5 grams of total fat, 3 grams of saturated fat. 1 percent milk has 2-1/2 percent of total fat and 1-1/2 grams of saturated fat. Skim milk is the best at 0 grams of fat. (Authors Anonymous: Health Notes, Your Health: 14, June 13, 1995). Skim milk has all the calcium and nutrients you need without the fat. In fact, skim milk has a slightly higher calcium content than whole milk.

When buying non-fat dry milk, buy the least expensive brand. It has the same nutrients as a more expensive brand. Just make sure it is fortified with vitamins A and D.

Researchers are saying loud and clear, unless a food is classified as being at least 97% fat-free, it is not considered a low-fat food. If you cannot find ground turkey or chicken that is at least 97% fat-free, buy turkey or chicken breasts that are classified as at least 97% fat-free. Have the breasts ground at the meat counter or grind it yourself.

Defatted soy flour can usually be purchased in health food stores and stores selling bulk foods. Use the phone to call different stores. If a store knows that you and others are interested in buying a certain product, they usually will stock it. After reading all the health benefits of defatted soy flour, it is worth the effort to find it and use it in your recipes.

Oyster sauce can be purchased in most grocery stores. It is a low sodium product compared to salt and has a nice flavor.

RECIPES

— DESSERTS —

AL FISHER'S SPECIAL PIE

Mix in a large bowl until blended
   3 cups dry milk (do not dilute)
   3 cups defatted soy flour
   2 teaspoons baking powder

Add the following to the mixed dry ingredients.
   3 eggs
   2-1/2 cups skim milk
   1/2 cup honey (tupelo honey is suggested)
   1 (29 oz.) can pure pumpkin
   1 (20 oz.) can crushed unsweetened pineapple
   1 cup chopped nuts (either walnuts or pecans)

Use a large wooden spoon to blend all ingredients. Mix until well blended. Lightly spray four 9" pie pans, using no-stick cooking spray. Divide mixture equally among the 4 pie tins. (I use glass pie plates.) Sprinkle ground cinnamon over the top of each pie. Use cinnamon to cover entire top of pie.

Bake at 350 degrees about 40 minutes or until center of pie is firm. When pies have cooled, cover each with plastic wrap and refrigerate. Pies will keep well in the refrigerator for 2 weeks. Pies may also be frozen.

For a different taste, other fruit may be added to the pie. When adding additional fruit, I usually add about 2 cups. Orange or pineapple juice may be substituted for skim milk.

This recipe contains: potassium, magnesium, calcium, zinc, biotin, boron, manganese, choline, inositol, copper, folic acid, soy protein vitamin A, vitamin D, vitamin E and the B vitamins, especially thiamine.

AL FISHER'S PUMPKIN ORANGE FRUIT PIE

Mix the following in a large bowl until blended.

4 cups defatted soy flour

4 cups dry milk (undiluted)

2 teaspoons baking powder

Add the following to the dry ingredients and mix until well blended.

3 eggs

3-1/2 cups orange juice (I use calcium fortified)

1 (29 oz.) can pure pumpkin

1 (20 oz.) can crushed pineapple

3 cups mixed fruit (fresh or frozen)

1/3 cup honey (I use tupelo)

2 cups chopped walnuts or pecans (optional)

Lightly spray 4 or 5 9-inch pie tins, using non-stick cooking spray. (I use the glass pie plates.) If you use the 5 pie tins instead of 4 pie tins, the pie will not be as thick. Your choice.

Divide the mixture evenly among the pie tins. Sprinkle cinnamon evenly over the top of the pies. Use enough cinnamon to cover entire top of the pie.

Bake at 350 degrees for about 35 to 40 minutes if using the five pie tins, a little longer if using the four pie tins. The center of the pie should be firm to the touch.

Pies keep well in the refrigerator for 2 weeks at least. To save space in the refrigerator, I put two pies on a shelf and then put an aluminum cookie sheet over the top of the 2 pies and then 2 more pies on top of the cookie sheet. Pies may also be frozen.

This recipe contains: potassium, magnesium, calcium, zinc, biotin, manganese, choline, inositol, copper, folic acid, soy protein, vitamin C, vitamin E, vitamin A, vitamin D and the B vitamins, especially thiamine.

Note: If you use canned fruit (in its own juice), add the juice to the recipe. The pies will have a different taste. If using the juice, measure the amount of juice and reduce the orange juice by the same amount.

APPLE CUSTARD

5 cups thinly sliced apples
cinnamon to cover apples
1 pound non-fat cottage cheese with pineapple
1 cup yogurt (I use homemade)
2 eggs
3 tablespoons margarine (low-fat in tub)
4 tablespoons honey (I use tupelo)
4 tablespoons corn starch
2 teaspoons vanilla extract
1-1/2 cups skim milk
1-1/2 cups dry non-fat milk

Put sliced apples in a lightly greased 9 x 13 inch pan. Sprinkle cinnamon over top of sliced apples, enough to cover the apples.

In a blender or food processor put the remaining ingredients and only blend until smooth. You could also blend the ingredients by hand in a large bowl. Pour mixture over the sliced apples. Bake at 350 degrees for 45 to 50 minutes. Refrigerate and serve cold.

This recipe contains: calcium, potassium, magnesium, boron, manganese, zinc, copper, chromium, flourine, and the B vitamins, especially B_{12}.

APPLE SNOW

2 (0.3 oz.) packages orange sugar-free gelatin
1-1/2 cups orange juice (I use calcium fortified.)
1 cup non-fat dry milk
4 egg whites
2 tablespoons of honey (I use tupelo honey)
2 large bananas sliced
1 cup applesauce (I use natural no sugar added)
2 tablespoons orange rind

In a saucepan mix the gelatin and the juice. Heat to dissolve, stirring constantly. Set aside.

Beat egg whites with a electric mixer until stiff peaks form. Gradually add the dry milk, honey and the sliced bananas and continue to beat until smooth. Fold into the gelatin mixture. Add the applesauce and the grated orange rind. Mix well. Put mixture into a 9 x 9 inch glass dish. Refrigerate until firm.

This recipe contains: calcium, potassium, magnesium, boron, manganese, zinc, iron, folic acid, vitamin C, vitamin A, vitamin D, and especially the B vitamins.

Note: Egg whites may be omitted from the recipe.

APPLE FRITTERS

3/4 cup whole wheat pastry flour
3/4 cup defatted soy flour
1/2 cup non-fat dry milk
1 egg
3 apples (large) cut into bite-size chunks
2 tablespoons honey (I use tupelo honey)
1-1/4 cups non-fat yogurt

Put dry ingredients in a large bowl and mix until blended. Add egg, honey and yogurt. Blend well. Fold in the apple chunks.

Spray skillet with non-stick cooking spray. Put about 1 tablespoon of mixture onto hot skillet.

Sprinkle cinnamon on top of each fritter. Cook until golden brown, turn fritter and sprinkle again with cinnamon. Cook until golden brown. Fritters are good both hot and cold.

This recipe contains: calcium, magnesium, potassium, copper, manganese, boron, zinc, chromium, lecithin and the B vitamins, especially B_1.

Note: I also use a fry pan with a cover and cook fritters as noted above. If you would like a larger fritter, you could drop a 2 tablespoon amount onto the griddle instead of 1 tablespoon.

CHERRY CREME DESSERT

1 cup yogurt (I use homemade)
1 cup fat-free cottage cheese

Blend above ingredients in blender until smooth.

2 (0.3 oz.) packages of sugar-free cherry jello
1 cup pineapple juice
2 cups cherries (or strawberries) (fresh or frozen) cut into
    bite sized pieces

In a saucepan put jello and pineapple juice and mix well. Heat to dissolve. Let cool and add blended yogurt and cottage cheese. Add the cherries. Put into a 7 x 11 inch dish and refrigerate until firm.

This recipe contains: calcium, potassium, zinc, manganese, boron, flourine, magnesium, copper, chromium, vitamin C and the B vitamins, especially B_{12}.

CHOCOLATE FUDGE

3 tablespoons cocoa or carob powder
3 tablespoons honey (I use tupelo honey)
2 tablespoons fat-free tub margarine
3 cups non-fat dry milk
1 cup yogurt (homemade preferred)
1 cup chopped walnuts or pecans

Put all the ingredients in a bowl except the yogurt. I use a wooden spoon to blend the ingredients. Add the yogurt and the nuts. Blend well into dry milk mixture. Form balls and put in a freezer bag. Freeze and serve.

This recipe contains: calcium, magnesium, potassium, folic acid, vitamin K, vitamin A, vitamin D, and the B vitamins.

PINEAPPLE CHEESE KUCHEN

1-1/2 cups whole wheat pastry flour
1/2 cup defatted soy flour
1/4 cup olive oil
1/2 teaspoon baking powder
2 tablespoons honey (I use tupelo)

In a large bowl mix the above ingredients. Lightly grease a 9 x 13 inch pan and pat in dough onto the bottom and sides of pan. Bake 350 degrees for 15 minutes. Remove from oven.

1 (20 oz.) can of crushed pineapple
1-1/2 cups skim milk
3/4 cup non-fat dry milk
2 cups non-fat cottage cheese
1 (8 oz.) package non-fat cream cheese
2 tablespoons cornstarch
3 tablespoons honey (I use tupelo)
2 egg yolks
2 egg whites

Over the top of the baked dough, spread the pineapple evenly.

In a blender or food processor, mix the rest of the ingredients except the egg whites. Blend. Whip the egg whites until stiff. Add to blended ingredients. Put mixture over the top of crushed pineapple. Bake at 350 degrees for an additional 35 to 40 minutes. Serve hot or cold.

This recipe contains: calcium, potassium, manganese, magnesium, copper, zinc, flourine, selenium, and the B vitamins, especially B_{12}.

Note: For a different taste do not whip the egg whites, just add the 2 eggs to the batter mixture.

PINEAPPLE RICE PUDDING

2 (1 oz.) packages instant sugar-free vanilla pudding
2 cups fat-free sour cream
2 cups pineapple juice
1 can crushed pineapple
3 cups cooked rice

In a bowl put the pudding mix and sour cream. Mix until well blended. Gradually add pineapple juice, crushed pineapple, and juice. Mix until well blended. Fold in cooked rice and blend. Put mixture in a covered bowl and refrigerate. Keeps well in refrigerator for a week. You could also make half the recipe.

This recipe contains: manganese, calcium, boron, chromium, potassium, magnesium, zinc, copper, selenium, flourine, and the B vitamins, especially B_{12}.

PUDDING DELITE

1 package instant sugar-free jello (orange)
1 cup orange juice

In a bowl mix jello and orange juice. Heat to dissolve. Let cool.

1 package instant sugar-free pudding mix (vanilla)
2 cups skim milk
2 cups non-fat cottage cheese

In a blender or food processor (or mixed by hand) blend the above ingredients and also add the cooled gelatin mixture. Blend until smooth. Chill in the refrigerator.

When serving, top with fruit or crushed walnuts.

This recipe contains: calcium, vitamin C, copper, potassium, chromium, and some B vitamins.

RICE BRAN COOKIES

3 tablespoons honey (I use tupelo honey)
3 tablespoons olive oil
3/4 cup yogurt
2 egg whites
1 egg
1-1/2 teaspoons vanilla extract
1 cup rice bran
1 cup dry oatmeal
1 cup defatted soy flour
3/4 cup non-fat dry milk
1 teaspoon baking powder
1 cup raisins
3/4 cup chopped pecans or walnuts

In a large bowl combine honey and oil. Add yogurt, egg, egg whites and vanilla extract, beat well. Blend the dry ingredients with the nuts in a separate bowl. After the dry ingredients are well blended, add to the liquid ingredients and blend well.

Drop by a teaspoon onto a lightly greased cookie sheet. Bake at 350 degrees for 10 to 12 minutes. Makes about two and one half dozen cookies.

This recipe contains: potassium, magnesium, calcium, boron, folic acid, iron, copper, zinc, chromium, choline, inositol, vitamin C, vitamin A, vitamin D, vitamin E, and the B vitamins, especially thiamine.

Note: rice bran can be purchased in most health stores and stores selling bulk foods.

ORANGE SHERBET

1 (6 oz.) can frozen orange juice concentrate
1-1/4 cup skim milk
1 cup non-fat dry milk
1 teaspoon orange extract

Mix the above ingredients in a food processor or blender. Can also be mixed by hand. Put into a freezer container and freeze. When serving, top with crushed walnuts.

This recipe contains: calcium, vitamin C, potassium, chromium, manganese, magnesium, and the B vitamins.

FROZEN YOGURT

1/4 cup orange juice
1 package sugar-free strawberry jello

Put the jello and orange juice in a pan. Mix and heat to dissolve the gelatin. You can also heat in the microwave.

2 cups yogurt (I use homemade)
2 cups sliced strawberries

Add above ingredients to cooled jello. Mix well and put into a freezer container and freeze. When serving frozen yogurt let set for about 10 to 15 minutes beforehand to soften.

This recipe contains: calcium, potassium, magnesium, beta-carotene, vitamin C, manganese, zinc, chromium, vitamin A, vitamin D, and the B vitamins.

– BREADS –

REFRIGERATOR BREAD

2 packages of rapid rise yeast
1/4 cup warm water

In a bowl mix warm water and yeast. Let set about 5 minutes to activate the yeast.

1 cup warm water
1 cup non-fat dry milk
1/4 cup olive oil
2 cups whole wheat flour
3/4 cup defatted soy flour
2 tablespoons honey (I use tupelo)

In a large bowl mix the above ingredients with a wire whip or wooden spoon. Add yeast mixture and mix until you have a soft dough. Cover bowl and put dough in refrigerator overnight.

Shape dough into 2 small loaves. Put into 2 lightly greased loaf pans. Cover top of loaf with a little olive oil. Let rise in a warm place for about 2 hours. Bake at 350 degrees for 30 to 35 minutes.

This recipe contains: potassium, magnesium, manganese, copper, calcium, selenium, chromium, zinc and the B vitamins.

Note: You can also make dinner rolls instead of bread. Half fill lightly greased muffin tins. Let rise in a warm place for 1 hour. Bake 350 degrees 20 to 25 minutes.

ORANGE BREAD

1 cup oats (quick cooking)
3/4 cup defatted soy flour
1-1/4 cups whole wheat pastry flour
1 cup non-fat dry milk
1/2 teaspoon nutmeg
1 tablespoon orange rind
2-1/2 teaspoons baking powder
1 cup yogurt (homemade preferred)
3 tablespoons honey (I use tupelo honey)
3 tablespoons canola or olive oil
1 egg
1/2 cup orange juice concentrate (thaw but do not dilute)
1/2 cup chopped walnuts or pecans

In a large bowl add the dry ingredients and mix well. Add yogurt, honey, oil, egg, and the orange juice concentrate. Mix all the ingredients with a large spoon. Continue to mix until the ingredients are well blended. Fold in the nuts. Put the mixture into a 9 x 5 x 3 inch pan. Bake at 350 degrees for about 40 to 50 minutes.

This recipe contains: potassium, magnesium, calcium, manganese, copper, iron, zinc, chromium, choline, lecithin, folic acid, vitamin A, vitamin D, vitamin C, vitamin E, vitamin K, and the B vitamins, especially thiamine.

OATMEAL MUFFINS

3/4 cup whole wheat pastry flour
3/4 cup non-fat dry milk
3/4 cup defatted soy flour
1-1/2 cups dry oats
1 cup rice bran
2 teaspoons baking powder
1 cup raisins
1 egg
1/2 cup chopped walnuts or pecans
2 tablespoons honey (I use tupelo honey)
3 tablespoons canola or olive oil
1-2/3 cups of yogurt (homemade preferred)

Mix the dry ingredients in a large bowl until well blended. Add the raisins and mix well. In a separate bowl mix the rest of the ingredients and blend well. Add to the dry ingredients and mix until well blended.

Fill about 12 lightly greased muffin tins. Bake at 350 degrees for about 20 to 25 minutes.

This recipe contains: potassium, magnesium, calcium, iron, zinc, copper, manganese, chromium, folic acid, choline, lecithin, vitamin E, vitamin A, vitamin D, vitamin K, and the B vitamins, especially thiamine.

Note: Rice bran and defatted soy flour can be purchased in stores selling bulk foods or in health stores. Tupelo honey can also be purchased in health food stores. To save time call the different stores in your area until you find one that stocks these foods. The health benefits you derive are worth the effort.

PINEAPPLE MUFFINS

1-1/2 cups dry oats
1 cup whole wheat pastry flour
1/2 cup defatted soy flour
1/2 cup non-fat dry milk
2 teaspoons baking powder (If using low-sodium baking
     powder, use 3 teaspoons)
2 eggs
1 cup crushed pineapple
3 tablespoons canola or olive oil
1-1/4 cups yogurt (homemade preferred)
1 cup chopped pecans or walnuts (optional)

Blend the dry ingredients in a bowl. Gradually add the yogurt and crushed pineapple. Mix well. Add the oil and eggs. Mix until the ingredients are well blended. If using the nuts, fold into the mixture. Fill lightly greased muffin tins 2/3 full. Bake at 350 degrees for about 25 to 30 minutes or until firm on top. Makes 12 muffins.

This recipe contains: potassium, magnesium, calcium, manganese, zinc, iron, copper, chromium, folic acid, lecithin, vitamin E, vitamin A, vitamin D, and the B vitamins.

Note: Whole wheat pastry flour can be purchased in stores selling bulk foods. It has the same vitamin content as whole wheat flour, but is a softer wheat and does not have the strong taste of whole wheat flour. I find that if a store does not carry it and they know you are interested in purchasing it, they will usually order it for you.

BANANA PANCAKES

2 eggs
1 cup of whole wheat pastry flour
1/2 cup defatted soy flour
1/2 cup of non-fat dry milk
1/2 teaspoon cinnamon
1 teaspoon cinnamon
1 teaspoon baking powder
1 tablespoon honey (I use tupelo)
2 bananas mashed (large)
1 cup non-fat sour cream

In a large bowl mix the above ingredients until smooth. Mixture can also be blended in the blender or food processor. Lightly spray griddle with no-stick cooking spray. Drop 2 tablespoons of the mixture on to the hot griddle and cook until golden brown on both sides.

This recipe contains: potassium, magnesium, calcium, copper, chromium, manganese, zinc, lecithin, vitamin A, vitamin D, and the B vitamins, especially B_1 and B_6.

COTTAGE CHEESE PANCAKES

3/4 cup defatted soy flour
1 teaspoon baking powder
1 cup non-fat cottage cheese
2 eggs
2 tablespoons canola or olive oil
1 tablespoon honey (I use tupelo)

Mix the above ingredients in a blender and whirl until smooth. Also can be mixed by hand in a large bowl with a wooden spoon.

Spray skillet with no-stick cooking spray. Put 2 tablespoons of mixture on skillet and cook until golden brown on both sides.

This recipe contains: potassium, magnesium, calcium, lecithin, zinc, copper, the B vitamins, especially B_1.

— APPETIZERS —

HUMMUS

1 (15 oz.) can of cooked chick-peas, drained
2 tablespoons of sesame seeds
1 tablespoon of lemon juice
2 tablespoons of yogurt
2 cloves of garlic, peeled and crushed
1/4 teaspoon of paprika
1/2 tablespoon of parsley
1/4 cup of minced scallions

Place sesame seeds in oven for 15 minutes at 350 degrees, until toasted brown. Place chick-peas in food processor, add sesame seeds and process of 1-2 minutes. Add lemon juice, yogurt, garlic and paprika and blend until smooth. Add and additional spices you feel will enhance the flavor. Consider mustard, cumin, corriander, basil.

This recipe contains: copper, magnesium, potassium, manganese, choline, zinc, vitamin E and the B vitamins.

KRISTIN'S PHYLLO SURPRISE

Phyllo dough sheets (can be purchased in frozen food section
   of most grocery stores)
mustard
imitation bacon bits
fat free shredded cheese or part skim mozzarella

Cut 4 x 8 inch slices from a sheet of defrosted phyllo dough. On each slice, spread a thin covering of mustard. Sprinkle bacon bits over mustard. Add a layer of shredded cheese. Wrap and pinch ends of dough to seal.

Bake at 415 degrees for about 10 minutes on cookie sheets sprayed with nonstick cooking spray.

Note: When selecting phyllo dough, note nutrition label. Get 0 Grams saturated fat.

SALMON DIP

1 (15 oz.) can salmon
1 (8 oz.) package fat-free cream cheese
1 teaspoon garlic powder
3 tablespoons dried parsley
1/2 cup finely chopped onion
1/2 cup finely chopped celery
1 tablespoon of salsa

Mix above ingredients in a bowl or in a blender / food processor. Try both ways. If mixed in the blender/food processor the dip will be smoother. A different taste!

This recipe contains: omega-3, calcium, potassium, selenium, flourine, magnesium, chromium, and iodine.

SALMON MOUSSE

1 (14 oz.) can of salmon
1 cup of yogurt
1 cup of non fat cottage cheese
1 packet of unflavored gelatin
1/4 cup of white wine
1/4 cup of dill
1/2 teaspoon of pepper

Mash salmon in a bowl. Place in a blender with yogurt, cottage cheese, and dill. Pour wine into a small pan and over low heat add gelatin until dissolved. Add to salmon, yogurt and cottage cheese and mix completely. Put mixture into a mold and chill 3-4 hours.

This recipe contains: omega 3 (thought to protect against heart disease), calcium, magnesium, potassium, iron, zinc, copper, inositol, vitamins A, D, E. K as well as the B vitamins.

TUNA MOUSSE - DIP AND SPREAD

2 cups non-fat cottage cheese
1 (8 oz.) package non-fat cream cheese
2 (6 oz.) cans solid white albacore tuna in water
1 cup finely chopped celery
1 cup finely chopped red onion
3 tablespoons chopped parsley (I use dried)
2 teaspoons garlic powder
1 tablespoon unflavored gelatin
1/4 cup orange juice

Put cottage cheese, cream cheese, and tuna in blender . Blend until smooth. Put into a bowl and add celery, onion, parsley and garlic powder. Mix well.

Mix gelatin and orange juice in a small pan. Let set for a few minutes to soften. Heat to dissolve. (I use the microwave.) Add gelatin to the other ingredients. Refrigerate several hours or overnight before serving. Delicious!

Serve with crackers. I look for the fat-free or reduced fat crackers. It also can be served with chopped vegetables.

This recipe contains: omega-3, selenium, chromium, calcium, magnesium, potassium, zinc, folic acid, iodine, beta-carotene, manganese, and B vitamins.

Note: Mousse can also be frozen. Solid pack white albacore tuna in water has more Omega-3 than chunk tuna.

– SOUPS –

CREAM OF BROCCOLI SOUP

2 cups chopped broccoli
3 cups chicken broth
1/2 cup chopped onion
2 cups skim milk
1 cup non-fat dry milk
1 teaspoon pepper
2 tablespoons corn starch

In a sauce pan cook broccoli and onion in chicken broth until soft. Puree in blender or food processor.

To contents in saucepan add skim milk, dry milk and pepper. Cook about 15 more minutes. Thicken with cornstarch dissolved in skim milk. Continue cooking until soup is slightly thickened.

This recipe contains: alpha-carotene, beta-carotene, calcium, magnesium, potassium, inositol, chromium, zinc, iron, folic acid, vitamin A, vitamin D, vitamin C, vitamin K, and the B vitamins.

CREAM OF MUSHROOM SOUP

2 cups mushrooms, chopped
1 medium onion, sliced
1 tablespoon oyster sauce
2 tablespoons defatted chicken broth

In a saucepan lightly sprayed with non-stick cooking spray, saute mushrooms and onions in the oyster sauce and chicken broth until tender. Set aside.

1/2 cup nonfat dry milk
1-1/2 cups defatted chicken broth
1 cup skim milk
2 tablespoons corn starch

In a blender or food processor put above ingredients with mushroom mixture. Blend until smooth. Return to saucepan and stir over medium heat until mixture has thickened.

This recipe contains: potassium, calcium, copper, chromium, manganese, magnesium and B_{12}.

CREAM OF PEA SOUP

2 cups peas (canned or frozen)
2 teaspoons light soy sauce or oyster sauce
1-1/2 cups evaporated skim milk
1 cup defatted chicken broth
1/2 cup nonfat dry milk
2 tablespoons corn starch
3 tablespoons dried onion

In a blender or food processor, put above ingredients except the dried onion. Blend until smooth.

Put all, including dried onion into a saucepan. Cook and stir over medium heat until soup has thickened. Serve hot.

This recipe contains: potassium, calcium, chromium, zinc, copper, manganese, iron, magnesium, and B vitamins, especially B_2 and B_{12}.

− YOGURT RECIPES −

MICROWAVE YOGURT

3 cups of non-fat dry milk
7 cups of skim milk
9 tablespoons of non-fat commercial yogurt

In a 2 quart microwave safe bowl put the dry milk. Gradually add the skim milk and mix until well blended. Put into the microwave and heat on high heat for 14 minutes or at 175 and 180 degrees if you have a temperature probe.

Remove from microwave. Put bowl on a hot-pad. Let cool until milk temperature is between 115 and 120 degrees. Leave bowl on hot-pad. Add the 9 tablespoons of commercial yogurt and blend well into milk mixture.

Leave the bowl on the hot-pad and set it in a warm place, away from drafts. Cover dish with a large towel. Let yogurt set for about 10 hours. The longer the yogurt is left to set, the thicker it will get. Put yogurt into containers (if desirable) with covers and refrigerate. You can add fruit or artificial sweeteners to your yogurt for a sweet taste before serving. It is also a good mixer for cold cereals. Experiment!

This yogurt has a much higher magnesium content than the yogurt purchased in the store because of the large amount of dry milk added to the recipe. It also increases the calcium and vitamin D content of the recipe. Your body will love the benefits it derives from this recipe. This recipe also contains vitamin K and the B vitamins.

Note: You could also save some yogurt from your previous recipe to use as a starter for your next batch of yogurt. It is not always necessary to use commercial yogurt as a starter.

YOGURT DRESSING

2 tablespoons light or fat-free mayonnaise
1 cup of yogurt (homemade preferred)
1 teaspoon spicy mustard
1 package artificial sweetener (sugar-free)

Mix above ingredients in a bowl. Put in a plastic container with a cover and refrigerate.

This recipe contains: calcium, potassium, magnesium, vitamin A, vitamin D, vitamin K, and the B vitamins.

– SALADS –

TUNA SALAD WITH YOGURT DRESSING

2 cans of solid pack tuna in water
1/2 cup chopped onion
1/2 cup chopped celery
3/4 cup chopped green or red pepper
1 medium tomato chopped

Put the tuna in a colander and rinse with cold water to reduce the sodium. Put tuna in a bowl and add the onion, celery, pepper, and the tomato. Mix well and add enough of the yogurt dressing to blend the mixture. Refrigerate the rest of the dressing and save for another salad.

This recipe contains: omega-3, potassium, magnesium, iron, beta-carotene, folic acid, zinc, vitamin C, vitamin K, and the B vitamins.

IMITATION CRAB MEAT SALAD

1 pound chopped imitation crab meat
1 cup chopped celery
1 cup chopped green or red pepper
1 medium red onion sliced thin
2 medium tomatoes chopped
yogurt dressing

Put imitation crab meat in a colander and rinse with cold water to reduce the sodium in it. Put crab meat into a large bowl and add the rest of the ingredients. Blend well. Add enough of the yogurt dressing to blend the ingredients, or to suit your taste. Yogurt dressing is listed in the contents of this book.

This recipe contains: potassium, calcium, magnesium, vitamin C, vitamin A, vitamin K, vitamin D, iron, beta-carotene, copper, zinc, and the B vitamins.

CRANBERRY SALAD

1 pound fresh cranberries chopped fine (I use a food
    processor or a blender)
1 (20 oz.) can crushed pineapple
1 cup chopped celery
3/4 cup chopped walnuts or pecans
1-1/2 cups sliced strawberries (fresh or frozen)
1-1/2 cups orange or pineapple juice
2 packages cherry gelatin (I use sugar-free gelatin)

In a sauce-pan put the gelatin and the orange or pineapple juice. Mix
and let set for a minute to soften. Heat to dissolve, stirring constantly. Do
not let boil. To the gelatin gradually add the cranberries, strawberries,
celery and the nuts. Blend well into the gelatin mixture. Put mixture into
a 8 x 12 inch glass dish. Refrigerate until firm.

This recipe contains: beta-carotene, vitamin C, manganese, potassium, magnesium, iron, zinc, calcium, and especially the B vitamins.

Note: When fresh cranberries are in the stores, I buy them and freeze
them. This way I have cranberries most of the year to make this salad.

PUMPKIN CREME SALAD

2 (0.3 oz.) packages orange sugar-free gelatin
2 cups orange juice (I use calcium fortified orange juice)
1 cup yogurt (I use homemade yogurt.)
1 (29 oz.) can pure pumpkin
1 (20 oz.) can crushed pineapple & juice
1 cup chopped walnuts or pecans

Put gelatin and orange juice in sauce pan. Heat to dissolve. Remove from heat and add yogurt. Blend with a wooden spoon. Add pineapple and pumpkin. Blend well and add nuts. Blend. Put into a 8 x 10 inch pan. Refrigerate.

This recipe contains: beta-carotene, alpha-carotene, calcium, magnesium, potassium, manganese, zinc, chromium, copper, boron, folic acid, vitamin C, vitamin A, vitamin D vitamin E, vitamin K and the B vitamins.

PUMPKIN CHEESE GELATIN SALAD

2 (0.3 oz.) packages orange sugar-free gelatin
1 cup orange juice (I use calcium-fortified)
1 cup of yogurt (homemade preferred)
3 tablespoons of honey (I use tupelo honey)
1 teaspoon of vanilla extract
1-1/2 cups of non-fat cottage cheese
1-1/2 cups of cooked pumpkin (or canned pumpkin)

In a saucepan put the jello, add the orange juice. Mix well and heat to dissolve the gelatin, stirring constantly. Puree the cottage cheese in a food processor or a blender. Add to the cooled orange gelatin. Add the rest of the ingredients and mix with a large spoon until well blended. Put into a 8 x 10 inch glass dish. Refrigerate until firm. Cut into squares and serve.

This recipe contains: beta-carotene, alpha-carotene, calcium, magnesium, potassium, iron, folic acid, vitamin C, vitamin A, vitamin D, vitamin K, and the B vitamins.

− FRUIT −

FLUFFY APRICOTS

Put one pound of whole dried apricots in a one quart bowl. You can use either a glass or plastic bowl with a cover. Cover with orange juice. Put the cover on the bowl. I use the calcium fortified orange juice. When using orange juice, why not get the benefit of calcium from the calcium fortified orange juice? Let the apricots set on the counter top overnight, then refrigerate for a gourmet treat!. Keep refrigerated until dish is empty. Guess what! You will like them enough to do this recipe over and over again.

This recipe is a good source of beta-carotene (vitamin A), potassium, iron, magnesium, calcium, vitamin C, vitamin P, vitamin K, and the B vitamins.

– MAIN DISHES –

STIR FRY TURKEY DINNER

1-1/2 pounds of turkey breasts (98% or 99% fat free)
1/2 cup of chopped green or red peppers
1/2 pound of tofu cut into 1/2 inch squares
1 cup of chopped celery
1 cup of sliced mushrooms
1 large onion sliced thin
2 cups of frozen peas thawed
2 tablespoons parmesan fat-free grated cheese
2 tablespoons olive oil
1 tablespoon oyster sauce
3 cups cooked brown rice

Cut the turkey breast into strips about 1/2 inches thick. Put turkey strips into a large fry pan or a wok. Add olive oil, sliced onions, sliced mushrooms, chopped celery, and chopped pepper. Cook on medium heat until turkey is lightly cooked.

Add tofu squares, oyster sauce. Cook until turkey is tender. Add thawed peas and parmesan cheese and continue to cook for 5 to 10 minutes longer. Serve over cooked brown rice.

This recipe contains: potassium, magnesium, iron, boron, chromium, tryptophan, calcium, vitamin C, vitamin E, beta-carotene, zinc, and the B vitamins, especially thiamine.

Note: Oyster sauce can be purchased in most food stores. You will enjoy the taste of oyster sauce in this recipe. When buying tofu, buy the kind that has been processed with calcium. Be a label reader. Most researchers are saying that meat or poultry should be no less than 97% fat-free to be low-fat. I try to buy turkey or chicken breasts that are 98% or 99% fat-free. I also look for 98% or 99% fat-free ground turkey. If I cannot find it, I have the turkey breasts ground at the meat counter or I grind it myself.

TURKEY VEGETABLE DINNER

1 cup thinly sliced potatoes
1 cup thinly sliced carrots
3/4 cup raw brown rice
3/4 cup thinly sliced red onion
1 pound of ground turkey or chicken browned (at least
    97% fat-free)
3 cups spaghetti sauce (low-fat)

Put ingredients in a lightly greased casserole in layers in order listed. Cover casserole. Bake at 350 degrees for 1 hour. Remove cover and continue to bake for 30 minutes more.

This recipe contains: potassium, magnesium, beta-carotene, alpha-carotene, copper, chromium, zinc, tryptophan, selenium, iron, vitamin C, and the B vitamins, especially B_{12} and B_1 (thiamine).

TURKEY HASH

1 pound ground turkey
2 cups cooked tomatoes
1 cup chopped celery
1 cup of cooked brown rice
1 cup onion chopped
1 cup green pepper
2 teaspoons chili powder
1 tablespoon oyster sauce

Brown ground turkey and then mix above ingredients with the browned turkey and put into a lightly greased 2 quart casserole. Bake at 350 degrees for 50 to 60 minutes.

This recipe contains: potassium, magnesium, iron, beta-carotene, tryptophan, chromium, and the B vitamins.

Note: This recipe may also be cooked in a crockpot at medium heat 4 to 5 hours.

TURKEY CASSEROLE

1 pound ground turkey (at least 97% fat-free)
1/2 cup chopped onion
1/2 cup chopped celery
1 (12 oz.) jar fat-free turkey gravy
1-1/2 cups mashed potato
1 cup fat-free cheddar cheese

In a skillet brown ground turkey, onions and celery. Lightly grease a 2 quart casserole then layer in the following order: browned turkey, onions and celery, gravy, mashed potatoes, cheddar cheese. Bake at 350 degrees for 25 to 30 minutes.

This recipe contains: potassium, calcium, copper, chromium, zinc, iron, manganese, tryptophan, magnesium and B vitamins.

PINEAPPLE TURKEY

2 pounds of boneless turkey breasts, cut into serving pieces
    (turkey should be at least 97% fat-free)
2 tablespoons canola or olive oil
2 tablespoons of oyster sauce
1 (20 oz.) can crushed pineapple
1 cup defatted chicken broth
1 tablespoon salsa
1 red onion sliced (medium)
cooked brown rice

Brown the turkey pieces in the oil in a skillet. Place the browned turkey pieces in a slow cooker. Put oyster sauce evenly over turkey pieces.

Combine crushed pineapple, salsa and chicken broth. Pour over turkey pieces. Cook 2 to 3 hours in slow cooker on high until turkey pieces are tender.

If you wish to thicken sauce, take some from slow cooker, put sauce in bowl and add 1 tablespoon of cornstarch. Return to cooker and cook until sauce is thickened. Serve over cooked brown rice.

This recipe contains: potassium, magnesium, manganese, copper, chromium, tryptophan, selenium, zinc, iron, vitamin E and especially the B vitamins.

ORANGE CHICKEN

3 pounds of boneless skinless chicken breasts
    cut in serving pieces
paprika
1 medium red onion, sliced
1-1/2 cups celery, chopped
1-1/2 cups carrots, chopped
2 tablespoons honey (I use tupelo honey)
1 (6 oz.) can frozen orange juice concentrate (thaw, but
    do not dilute)

Sprinkle chicken breasts with paprika. In the bottom of a slow cooker (crockpot) place onions, celery, and carrots in layers. Then place chicken breasts on top. Over top of the chicken breasts put the orange juice concentrate that has been mixed with the tupelo honey. Cover pot and turn the slow-cooker to high and cook about 2-1/2 hours. Then turn slow-cooker to medium and cook until chicken is tender about 2 to 3 hours more.

This recipe contains: potassium, magnesium, beta-carotene, alpha-carotene, vitamin C, zinc, iron, copper, selenium, calcium, and especially the B vitamins.

STUFFED GREEN PEPPERS

6 green peppers
1/2 pound ground turkey (at least 97% fat-free)
1/4 cup chopped onion
3 tablespoons chopped pimento
1 cup cooked rice
1 tablespoon oyster sauce or low-sodium soy sauce
1 can cream mushroom soup (98% fat-free)
1 teaspoon prepared mustard

Cut a slice off the top of each pepper. Remove core, seeds and white membrane. Stand peppers upright in a crockpot. In a bowl combine all the ingredients except the soup and mustard. Spoon mixture into the 6 peppers. Combine soup and mustard and put over the top of the stuffed peppers.

Cover the pot and set on low. Cook for 8 to 10 hours.

This recipe contains: potassium, magnesium, chromium, manganese, selenium, copper, calcium and B vitamins.

SALMON POTATO CASSEROLE

4 cups mashed potatoes
1 cup cooked peas
1 (15 oz.) can salmon
1 can cream of mushroom soup (98% fat-free)

Put mashed potatoes in a lightly greased 2 quart casserole leaving a deep hollow in the center. In a bowl mix the remaining ingredients. Put the salmon mixture in the center (deep hollow) of the mashed potatoes. Bake 350 degrees for 30 to 40 minutes.

This recipe contains: omega-3, calcium, potassium, magnesium, selenium, chromium, iodine, manganese, copper, iron, zinc and B vitamins.

SALMON PUFF

1 (15 oz.) can salmon
1-1/2 cups bread crumbs (I use whole wheat)
1/2 cup defatted soy flour
2 eggs
1-1/2 cups shredded fat-free cheddar cheese
1 cup sliced onions
2 tablespoons corn starch
2 teaspoons oyster sauce
3/4 cup yogurt
1-1/4 cups skim milk
3/4 cup dry non-fat milk powder
1/2 teaspoon dry mustard
2 tablespoons of light margarine (I use tub margarine)

Lightly grease a 8 x 12 inch pan. Flake salmon including bones. Put layers in the following order: salmon, bread crumbs, cheddar cheese, onions.

In a bowl mix the remaining ingredients. Put over top of layers. Dot top with margarine. Bake at 350 degrees for 35 to 40 minutes or until top is lightly browned.

This recipe contains: omega-3, calcium, potassium, flourine, selenium, magnesium, chromium, iodine, manganese, copper, vitamin E, vitamin A, vitamin D, and the B vitamins, especially vitamin B_{12}.

TUNA CASSEROLE

3/4 cup chopped red or green pepper
3/4 cup chopped red onion
1 tablespoon canola or olive oil
1 can cream of mushroom soup (98% fat-free)
1/2 cup non-fat dry milk
3 tablespoons skim milk
2 (6-1/2 oz.) cans tuna solid pack in water drained
1-1/2 cups frozen peas
cooked brown rice

In a 2 quart microwave safe bowl put oil, peppers and onion. Microwave on high for 3 minutes. You could also cook in a skillet on top of the stove until peppers and onion are tender.

Blend in soup, dry milk, skim milk, peas, and tuna broken into bite size pieces. Cook in microwave on high for about 12 minutes. You could also bake in oven at 350 degrees for 30 to 35 minutes. Serve over cooked brown rice.

This recipe contains: omega-3, calcium, magnesium, potassium, copper, zinc, iron, beta-carotene, folic acid, vitamin C, vitamin E, and the B vitamins, especially thiamine.

Note: Stores are now selling canned soups that are 98% fat free. They taste very good and you are eating a healthy food to benefit your body.

HALIBUT STEAK CASSEROLE

2 pounds halibut steak cut into serving pieces
dash of tabasco sauce rubbed into each piece of halibut
1 cup chopped red or green pepper
3/4 cup chopped celery
1 clove garlic minced
2 tablespoons olive or canola oil
1 (28 oz.) can tomatoes
1/2 cup non-fat dry milk
1/4 cup minced parsley
1 tablespoon honey (tupelo preferred)

In a 2 quart microwave safe dish combine celery, peppers, onions, garlic, and parsley. Cook in microwave on high for 3 minutes or cook on top of stove in a skillet until vegetables are tender.

Remove vegetables from casserole and put the halibut steaks on bottom of dish. To the tomatoes add the dry milk and the cooked vegetables. Put over the halibut steaks. Cook in microwave on high for about 9 minutes or until fish flakes easily with a fork.

The casserole can also be baked in the oven at 350 degrees for 25 to 30 minutes.

This recipe contains: omega-3, beta-carotene, iron, zinc, potassium, magnesium, calcium, folic acid, vitamin C, vitamin E, and the B vitamins, especially B_1, B_2, B_6, and B_{12}.

CHILI CON CARNE

1 pound ground turkey (at least 97% fat-free)
3/4 cup chopped onion
3/4 cup chopped celery
3/4 cup chopped green or red pepper

Put above ingredients in a 10 inch skillet. Heat, stirring until ground turkey is cooked.

1 quart spaghetti sauce (low-fat)
1 tablespoon chili powder
1 teaspoon paprika
2 (15-1/2 oz.) cans kidney beans

Add above ingredients to the turkey mixture. Simmer over low heat for about 40 minutes.

This recipe contains: magnesium, potassium, zinc, iron, chromium, copper, manganese, beta-carotene, tryptophan, calcium, and the B vitamins.

EASY OVEN PIZZA

1 pound ground turkey (at least 97% fat-free)
1 cup chopped onion
1/2 cup chopped green or red peppers

In a skillet with a tablespoon of olive oil brown the above ingredients.

Lightly grease a 9 x 13 inch pan and put the browned turkey, onions and peppers on the bottom. Add the spaghetti sauce and mushrooms.

2 cups low-fat spaghetti sauce
3/4 cup chopped mushrooms (optional)

Mix the following and put over the turkey mixture.

2 eggs
1 cup skim milk
1 tablespoon olive oil
1 cup flour (your choice whole wheat or white)
1 teaspoon baking powder

Top with shredded cheese (3/4 cup fat-free shredded cheddar cheese or part-skim mozzarella).

Bake at 375 degrees for 30 to 35 minutes.

This recipe contains: potassium, magnesium, calcium, iron, zinc, copper, chromium, beta-carotene, manganese and B vitamins.

– VEGETABLES –

STIR FRY CABBAGE

3 cups finely shredded cabbage
3/4 cup chopped green or red pepper
3/4 cup chopped green onions
2 tablespoons olive oil
2 tablespoons vinegar
3 tablespoons low sodium soy sauce
1 teaspoon dill
1-1/2 tablespoons honey (I use tupelo honey)
1/3 cup defatted soy flour

In a wok or a fry pan add all the above ingredients except the defatted soy flour. Stir-fry until the vegetables are lightly cooked. In a small bowl add some of the liquid from the vegetables to the soy flour. Mix and then add to the vegetables to thicken. Serve hot.

This recipe contains: beta-carotene, potassium, magnesium, calcium, iron, manganese, zinc, chromium, lecithin, copper, vitamin E, vitamin K, vitamin C, and the B vitamins, especially thiamine.

SWEET POTATO PIE

1 pound of ground turkey (at least 97% fat-free)
3 cups cooked and mashed sweet potatoes
1 cup chopped celery
1 cup of chopped onion (red onion preferred)
2 tablespoons fat-free parmesan cheese
2 teaspoons low-sodium soy sauce
3 tablespoons margarine (I use tub margarine)
1/2 cup of part skim mozzarella cheese shredded

In a large fry pan add margarine, celery, onions, ground turkey and soy sauce. Simmer about 15 minutes or until ground turkey is lightly browned. Add the shredded cheese and sweet potatoes. Mix well. Put into a lightly greased 2 quart casserole. Sprinkle parmesan cheese over top of casserole. Bake at 350 degrees for about 30 to 35 minutes. Serves 4 to 6 people.

This recipe contains: beta-carotene, magnesium, potassium, calcium, zinc, copper, iron, folic acid, vitamin C, Vitamin E, and the B vitamins, especially thiamine.

Note: Always buy ground turkey that is at least 97% fat-free. Researchers are saying it is not low fat unless it is at least 97% fat-free.

SWEET POTATO CASSEROLE

2 cups of sweet potatoes cooked and mashed
3/4 cup of yogurt (I use homemade)
1/4 cup margarine (tub low-fat)
2 tablespoons honey (I use tupelo honey)
1 egg yolk
3 egg whites stiffly beaten

In a large bowl put the mashed sweet potatoes. Add the yogurt, margarine and egg yolk. Mix well and fold in the stiffly beaten egg whites. Put into a lightly greased casserole. Bake at 350 degrees for about 35 to 40 minutes.

This recipe contains: beta-carotene, calcium, potassium, copper, iron, folic acid, niacin, manganese and the B vitamins.

ZUCCHINI SOUFFLE

2-3/4 cups grated zucchini
1/3 cup whole wheat pastry flour
1/3 cup defatted soy flour
2 teaspoons cinnamon
1 cup shredded fat-free cheddar cheese
1/2 cup fat-free parmesan cheese
1 cup dry skim milk powder
1/4 cup olive or canola oil
1 cup chopped celery
1 cup chopped green or red pepper
1 cup chopped onion
3 eggs
2 tablespoons honey (tupelo)
1-1/2 cups yogurt (homemade)
1-1/2 cups skim milk

In a large bowl mix the dry ingredients and the cheddar cheese. Gradually add the remaining ingredients and mix until well blended. Put mixture in to a lightly greased 9 x 13 inch pan. Bake at 350 degrees about 50 minutes or until zucchini mixture is firm.

For a different taste you can also sprinkle extra cinnamon over top of casserole before baking. You can also add the egg yolks separately to the recipe. Then whip the egg whites until stiff and fold into the batter before baking.

This recipe contains: calcium, manganese, folic acid, beta-carotene, potassium, copper, zinc, iron, magnesium, vitamin E, vitamin A, vitamin D, and especially the B vitamins.

BIBLIOGRAPHY

Abraham, A. (1990). Magnesium is safe in reduction of incidents of arrhythmias, *Journal of Magnesium* 9: 177.

Abraham, G.E., & Grewal, H. (1990). A total dietary program emphasizing magnesium instead of calcium in the treatment of Osteoporosis, *Journal of Reproductive Medicine* 35: 503-507.

Abraham, G.E. (1991). The importance of magnesium in management of primary post-menopausal osteoporosis, *Journal of Nutritional Medicine* 2: 165-178.

Aldercreutz, H., Fotsis T., & Bannwart, C. (1986). Wahala: Determination of urinary lignans and phytoestrogen metabolites, potential antiestrogen and anticarcinogens in urine of women on various habitual diets, *Steroid Biochem* 25: 791-797.

Aldercreutz, H., Fotsis, T., Bannwart, C., & Brunow, C. (1991). Hose TA: Isotope dilution gas chromatographic-mass spectrometric method of the determination of lignans and isoflavonoids in human urine, including identification of genistein, *Chin Chim Acta* 199: 263-278.

Anderson, J.W., Johnstone, B.M., & Cook-Newell, M.E. (1995). Meta-analysis effects of soy protein intake on serum lipids, *New England Journal of Medicine* 333: 276-286.

Author Anonymous: Weight loss and yogurt keep you clear of cataracts (1996). *Natural Healing Newsletter* 8 (89): 8.

Authors Anonymous: Alpha carotene versus beta carotene (1990). *Journal National Cancer Institute* 81,21:1649.

Authors Anonymous: *American Journal of Dentistry* (1992). 5: 269.

Authors Anonymous: *Archives of Internal Medicine* 151, 3: 593.

Authors Anonymous: ESHA Research (Jan./Feb. 1995). Salem, Oregon. *Nutrition Action Healthletter.*

Authors Anonymous: *Health Notes, Your Health* (June 13, 1995). 14

Authors Anonymous: *Nutrition Action Healthletter,* Jan./Feb. 1995.

Authors Anonymous: Thiamine in Alzheimer's disease, *Annals of Neurology* (1990). 28-(2): 203-301.

Authors Anonymous: University of Texas *Lifetime Health Letter,* September, 1994.

Authors Anonymous: Vitamin C, *Consumer Reports on Health:* March, 1994.

Authors Anonymous, University of California at Davis, School of Medicine: Calcium, vitamins and other minerals in yogurt, *International Journal of Immunotherapy* 7: 205-210, 1992.

Authors Anonymous, University of Illinois: Heat releases beta-carotene and protein better than chewing does, (January, 1995). METLIFE, *Health Beat Bulletin* 2 (1).

Bariscoe, M., Ragen, C. (1966). Relation of magnesium on calcium metabolism in man, *American Journal of Nutrition* 19: 296.

Barnes, S. et al: (1994). Soy creates compound genistein, *Science News* 137: 19.

Block, G. et al: (1992). Fruits and vegetables cancer protection - A review of the epidemiological evidence, *Nutrition and Cancer,* 18 (1).

Block, G. (July 13, 1993). Vitamin C and cancer, your health.

Bruce, G.E. (1994). Nutrition and eye disease of the elderly, *Journal of Nutritional Biochemistry* 5: 66-76

Butterworth, C. Jr et al: (1992). Folate deficiency and cervical dysplasia, *Journal of American Medical Association* 267: 528-533.

Butterworth, R.F., & Besard, A.M. (1990). Thiamine-dependent enzyme changes in temporal cortex of patient with Alzheimer's disease, *Metal Brain Dis* 5: 179-184.

Carroll, K.K. (1991). Review of clinical studies on cholesterol-lowering response to soy protein, *Am Diet Assoc* 9: 820-827.

Cohen, L., & Kitzes, R. (1991). Infrared spectroscopy and magnesium content of bone mineral in osteoporotic women, *Israel Journal of Medical Science* 17: 1123.

Cox, I., Campbell, J., & Dowson, D. (1991). Red blood cell, magnesium and chronic fatigue syndrome, *Lancet* 337: 757-760, 1991

Fisher, R.C. (1989). *Osteoporosis, My High Calcium, Low Cholestorol Diet:* 7.

Fisher, R.C. (1992). *Research and Recipes on Osteoporosis, Heart Disease and Cancer:* 12-13.

Haas, R.H. (1988). Thiamine and the brain, *Annu Rev Nutr* 8: 483-515.

Hall, R. (June 25, 1973). *Journal of the American Medical Association.*

Hallfrisch, J. (1994). High plasma vitamin C associated with high plasma HDL and Cholostoral, *American Journal of Clinical Nutrition* 60:100-105.

Hilton, E. (1992). Yogurt can be an effective treatment for vaginal C. albicans infections, *Annals of Internal Medicine* 116: 353-357.

Hoffer, A., M.D., Ph.D. (1989). Orthomolecular medicine for physicians, New Canaan, Conn.: *Keats Publishing, Inc.*

Horwitt, M.K. et al: (1948). Investigations of human requirements of B-Complex vitamins, *National Research Bulletin* 116.

Kahn, J. (May 18, 1995). Low Ionized magnesium linked to migraine headaches, *Medical Tribune:* 7.

Mayne, S.T., Ph.D. (January 5, 1994). et al: Lung cancer in nonsmokers, *Journal of the National Cancer Institute.*

Meador, K., Loring, D., Nichols, M., Zanrini, E., Rivner, M., Posas, H., Thompson, E., & Moore, E. 1993. Preliminary findings of high-dose thiamine in dementia of Alzheimer's type, *Journal of Geriatrics, Psychiatry, & Neurology* 6: 222-229.

Meador, K.J., Nichols, M.E., Franke, P., Durkin, M.U., Oberzan, R.L., Moore, E.E., & Loring, D.W. (1993). Evidence for a central cholinergic effect of high-dose thiamine in dementia of Alzheimer's type disease, *Annals of Neurology* 34 (5): 724-726.

Murray, F. (May, 1990). Alzheimer's treatment & causes, *Better Nutrition:* 11.

Murray, F. (November 18, 1992). Compounds found in edible plants may increase resistance to breast and ovarian cancer, *Better Nutrition* 18.

Murray, F. (November 1989). The ups and downs of potassium levels, *Better Nutrition:* 18.

Nolan, K.A., Black, R.S., & Sheu, K.F.R. (1991). Trial of thiamine in Alzheimer's type disease, *Archives of Neurology* 48: 81-83.

Orey, C. (March, 1994). Natural beauty 20 secrets to eternal youth, *Let's Live.*

Pauling, L. (1993). Vitamin C strengthens immune system and destroys cancer cells, national cancer institute conference. *Linus Pauling Institute of Science and Medicine* 440: Page Mill Road, Palo Alto CA 94306.

Rath, M., M.D: Today's breakthroughs: tomorrow's cures, research summary, Matthias Rath, M.D., *Health Now,* 387 Ivy Street, San Francisco, CA 94102.

Reichman, M., Hayes et al: Vitamin A and subsequent development of prostate cancer, *First National Health and Nutrition Examination Survey,* Epidemiologic Follow-Up Study, Cancer Research 50: 2311-2315, 1990.

Reid, I., Ames, R., Evans, M., Gamble, D., & Sharpe, S. (1993). Increasing ability to absorb calcium, *New England Journal of Medicine* 328: 833.

Salmon, D.P., Thal, L.U., Butters, N., & Heidel, W.C. (1995). Low folic acid levels - high homocysteine levels may be risk for heart disease, *New England Journal of Medicine* 332: 286.

Schwartz, J. (1994). Vitamin C important anti-oxidant that directly neutralizes free radicals and is part of glutathione peroxidase pathway for repairing oxidative lipid membrane, *Journal of Clinical Nutrition* 59: 110-114.

Seelig, M.S. (1990). Increased magnesium need with use of combined estrogen and calcium for Osteoporosis, *Magnesium Research* 3: 197-215.

Seelig, M.S. (1964). The requirement of magnesium by the normal adult, *American Journal of Clinical Nutrition* XIV: 342.

Singh, R.B. (1990). A high-fat diet can steal both magnesium and calcium, *Journal Magnesium* 9: 255.

Stendig-Lindberg, G., M.D. (July 22, 1993). *Medical Tribune.*

Wahlquist, M.L. (1990). FRACP: Soy mimics female hormone estrogen, *British Medical Journal* 301: 905-6.

Young, V., & Scrimshaw, S. (1994). Soybean protein is capable of supporting body's need for amino acids, *American Journal of Clinical Nutrition* 59: SS, 12035-12125.

Zaman, Z., Roche, S., & Fielder, P. et al: (1992). Plasma concentrations of Vitamin A and E carotenoids in Alzheimer's disease, *Age & Aging* 21: 91-94.